T5T The Five Tibetan Exercise Rites

Carolinda Witt developed T5T over a period of five years and has since taught over 700 students and 25 teachers. With input from highly qualified health practitioners and the living laboratory of her own classrooms, she created a unique step-by-step program that gives people's bodies time to develop strength and flexibility. Knowing how most people restrict their breathing capacity and thereby vitality, she incorporated energy breathing and simple relaxation methods into T5T. The result is a daily dose of well-being that takes just 10 minutes a day. Carolinda is currently implementing her Teacher Training programs worldwide as T5T continues to grow and the demand for qualified teachers increases.

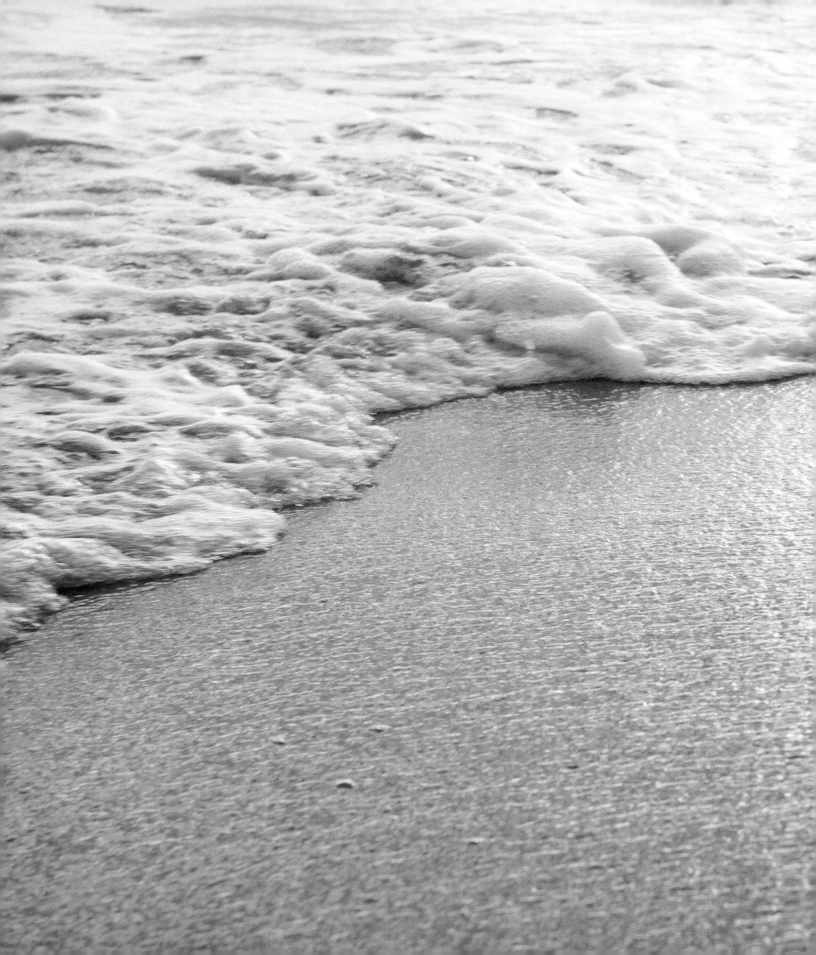

CAROLINDA WITT

The 10-Minute Rejuvenation Plan

T5T: The Revolutionary Exercise Program That Restores Your Body and Mind

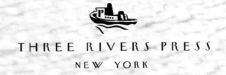

THREE RIVERS PRESS
NEW YORK

T5T is a registered trademark.

Three Rivers Press and the Tugboat design are registered trademarks of Random House, Inc.
Originally published in paperback in Australia as *T5T: The Five Tibetan Exercise Rites* by the Penguin Group
(Australia), a division of Pearson Australia Group Pty Ltd, in 2005.
Library of Congress Cataloging-in-Publication Data is available upon request.

ISBN: 978-0-307-34717-6
Printed in China

Design by John Canty © Penguin Group [Australia]

10 9 8 7 6 5 4 3 2 1

First U.S. Edition

T5T is simple, practical, effective and certainly mind/body altering. If you would love to become rejuvenated, remain calm, feel more vitality, be more flexible and simply look your absolute best, then now there is a new way to experience a greater state of well-being that takes just minutes a day, but lasts a lifetime. Dr. John F. Demartini, bestselling author of *The Breakthrough Experience*

I never thought it would be possible to gain more energy and become more relaxed in only ten minutes a day. But T5T manages just that. Amazing. Paul Wilson, bestselling author of *The Little Book of Calm*

Users of this book will build up strength and flexibility if they follow Carolinda's graded step-by-step plan—with mastery of each stage an essential goal before moving on to the next level of difficulty. The sections on breathing and core stability are a vital part of this program. The instructions are very clear and the use of many photographs makes this book easy to follow and a pleasure to use. Susie Lapin, physiotherapist

CONTENTS

3

RITES

4

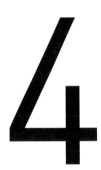

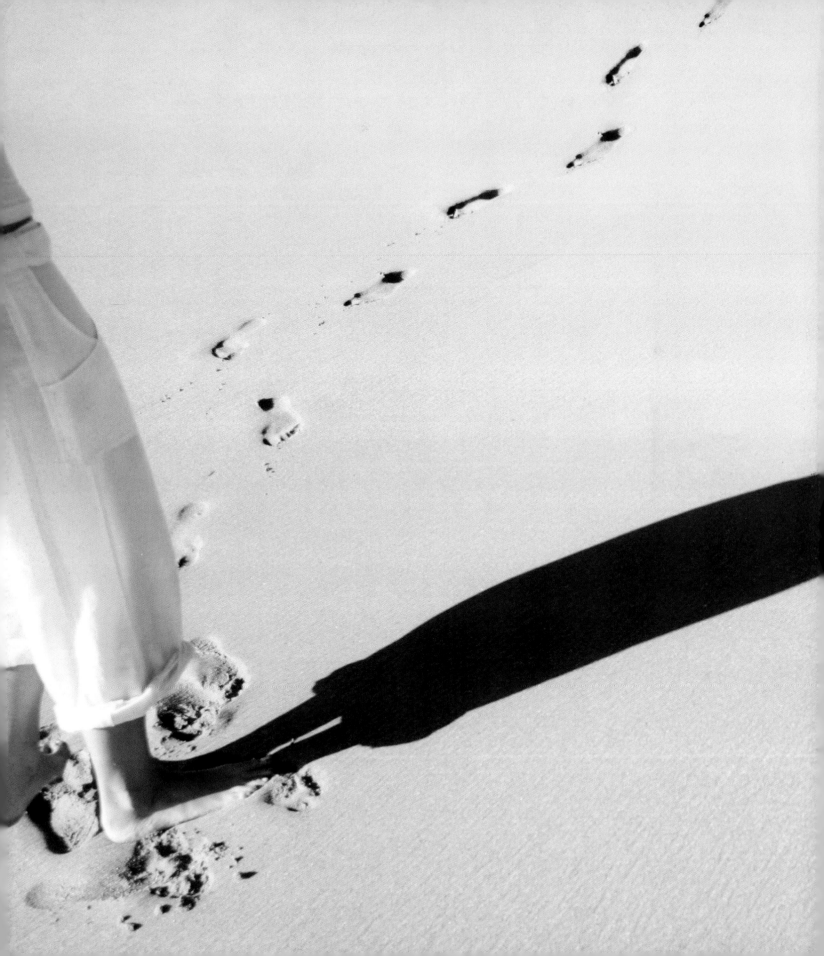

... in the end, it's not the years in your life, it's the life in your years.
Abraham Lincoln

We are all aging. From the moment we are born, we begin to age.

Time is catching up with the Forever Young generation, and we are waking to the reality that, unbelievably, we too are running out of time. Those first gray hairs, the stiffness in the morning as we get out of bed, the loss of libido and thereby potency in life—all these signs of aging ring alarm bells.

But our attitude toward aging is changing. We are challenging the view that to age is to become physically and mentally decrepit, a burden on our families and on society.

Because of today's increased life expectancy, the question we are now asking is "How do we remain younger, and healthier, longer?"

In our search for the legendary "fountain of youth" we are taking up exercise routines in ever increasing numbers, sometimes for the first time in our lives. With a growing interest in diet, nutritional supplementation and meditation, we are doing whatever we can to "stop the clock."

This search for the fountain of youth is illustrated in the legend of Shangri-La, a mystical place where people did not grow old but remained in an extended state of healthy youthfulness. The legend was the subject of *Lost Horizon*, a novel by James Hilton that was published in 1933 and made into an Oscar-winning movie in 1937. Shangri-La was fiction—or was it?

Also in the 1930s, in a separate but possibly related incident, a retired British Army officer called Colonel Bradford discovered a monastery in Tibet where the monks were remarkably old yet appeared healthy and "ageless." Colonel Bradford studied the five yoga postures carried out by the monks daily and brought them back to the West, where they became known as the Five Tibetan Rites of Rejuvenation. The Rites are still being practiced today.

The birth of T5T

I was introduced to the Five Tibetan Rites of Rejuvenation five years ago by a friend, a teacher of the Tibetan Rites. I was at a low point in my life, a kind of "crossroads crisis," and looking for new ways of being. When I began to practice the Five Rites, I felt as though the missing piece to a puzzle had slotted into place.

I felt better within myself than I had for years. My mind became calm. My backache completely disappeared, my skin glowed and my eyes sparkled. I felt strong and supple once again, with a newfound sense of purpose and well-being.

I was thrilled that the Five Rites took just 10 minutes of my busy day, yet I was experiencing such significant benefits.

After I had been practicing the Five Rites for six months, my family experienced a traumatic incident that resulted in the loss of a young and vital teenager. There were days when my body was so heavy with grief that I could barely carry out the Five Rites. I persevered because every time I finished my practice I felt

Yoga is a light; which, once lit, will never dim. The better your practice, the brighter the flame. BKS Iyengar

like my body had shed a ton of weight. My mind became centered, calm and clear. I truly believe that the Rites provided me with an internal rod of strength to lean on during that distressing time in my life. I've never stopped practicing the Five Rites, and I don't believe I ever will.

My friend who had taught me the Five Rites asked me to join her in teaching them in Sydney. We found that many people were interested in learning the Rites, and our classes became increasingly popular.

While I noticed that many students obtained amazing results, I also became aware that others were struggling beyond their capabilities, despite all advice to "go at their own pace." Inevitably, these people experienced muscle discomfort and even pushed themselves to the point of pain.

I began to envisage a way of adapting the Rites that would make them simpler and easier, so that more people would be able to make the 10-minute exercises a part of their lives. I took into account how different our modern sedentary lifestyle is from that of the monks, who would have most likely practiced the Rites from an early age. My solution was to blend the original ancient Rites with modern, Western techniques.

The result is T5T (The Five Tibetans), a completely new and much safer way of practicing the original rites.

A blend of ancient and modern methods, T5T combines the best of both worlds; it retains the integrity of the ancient rites, but improves core stability and strength by using modern methods to isolate certain muscle groups. The program is equally suited to those who are new to exercise and those who wish to increase their tone, flexibility, energy and well-being. T5T is a complete mind and body approach to physical development, calming your mind and improving your body tone and general health.

In developing the program I consulted highly qualified health practitioners who contributed their knowledge as well as ideas and inspiration. From **physiotherapy** and **Pilates** I incorporated the use of deep core stability muscles to support, strengthen, and protect the spine. From **chiropractic**, **osteopathy**, **Feldenkrais** and **occupational therapy**, I incorporated modifications and adaptations that would not only support and protect the whole body, but also encourage awareness of movement while practicing the postures and during normal life. Michael Grant White, "The Breathing Coach," contributed to T5T's approach to **breathing**. Finally, from the vast wisdom of **yoga** I incorporated the Complete Yogic Breath. Many of the tips on how to practice the postures also come from yoga.

I began by teaching my new method to some of my friends. They all experienced the immediate benefits I had been accustomed to seeing in earlier workshops, but they achieved them without strain. Realizing there was a genuine need for more people to achieve similar benefits, I developed a teaching workshop.

We know that the average person reaches peak respiratory function and lung capacity in their midtwenties. Then they begin to lose between 10 percent and 27 percent of respiratory capacity every decade! Unless you are doing something to maintain or improve your breathing capacity, it will decline, along with your health, appearance, life expectancy, and your emotional and spiritual well-being. **Michael Grant White (The Breathing Coach), founder of Optimal Breathing**

In developing my workshops I took the concept two steps further, focusing on breathing and relaxation techniques. My first step was to integrate a system of energy-inducing breathing into the program. For many years, I had utilized the power of the breath through practicing *pranayama* (breath control) and meditation. I had also studied various breathing techniques to assist me to get in touch with and release repressed emotions. I had used these methods successfully, both personally and with my clients in my natural therapies clinic, and knew what a powerful role breathing plays in any exercise program.

I also knew that most people take breathing for granted—a great mistake, as breath *is* life. Just like our other muscles, our respiratory muscles become weaker when they are not fully utilized. The maxim If you don't use it, you lose it! is really true.

By combining "energy" breathing exercises with the movements, my aim was to create a simple, short, daily routine that people could achieve and *enjoy*. T5T's Energy Breathing does just that—it provides more life energy to the body. It greatly assists in removing toxins and impurities as well as supplying life-enhancing oxygen to the body. It helps to calm and clarify the mind. When Energy Breathing is combined with the Five Tibetan Rites, the result is a very powerful yet easy way to perform yoga program that will maximize your ability to remain younger, fitter and healthier longer. Yet it takes only 10 to 15 minutes per day.

To maximize the benefits of the movements and the breathing in T5T, I included two powerful and enjoyable relaxation techniques. Centered on breathing, these methods help you to develop the ability to remain fully in the present, and achieve a very deep state of calm. They can also be used for meditation.

The growth of T5T

I have since taught more than 700 people in a rapidly expanding series of workshops around Australia and am now expanding internationally. I also teach T5T to individuals, companies and private groups. With T5T becoming more and more popular, more teachers are needed and I have developed a Teacher Training Program, which is currently under way.

Having taught so many students, I am well aware of the common mistakes that students can make. My unique method makes it easy for people to learn, taking them from Beginners through Intermediate to Advanced and beyond. This method has been tried and tested many times by students in my workshops, and it works.

My method is covered in this book, accompanied by photographs that illustrate the do's and don'ts of each posture. These photographs make it easy for you to get T5T right the first time.

Once learned, T5T will be yours for life. You will be able to practice the movements anywhere, and at any time. You won't have to waste time traveling to gyms or clubs, and you won't need any special equipment. Most important, T5T won't keep costing you money.

This book will enable you to experience what T5T has already achieved for hundreds of others.

•

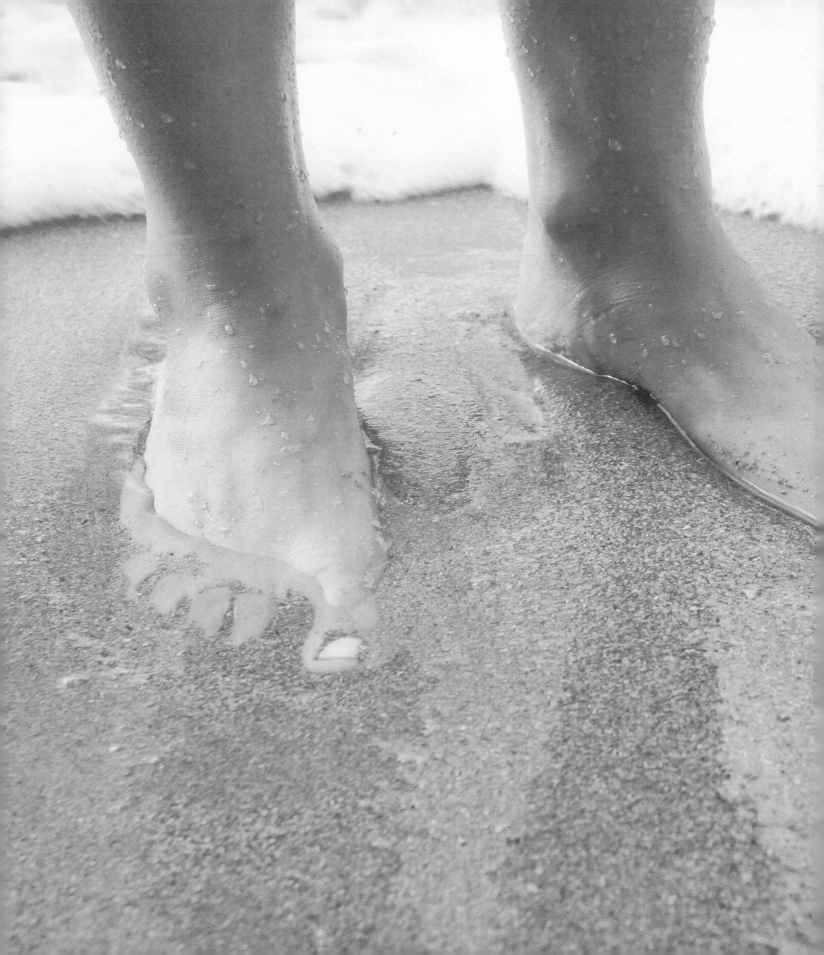

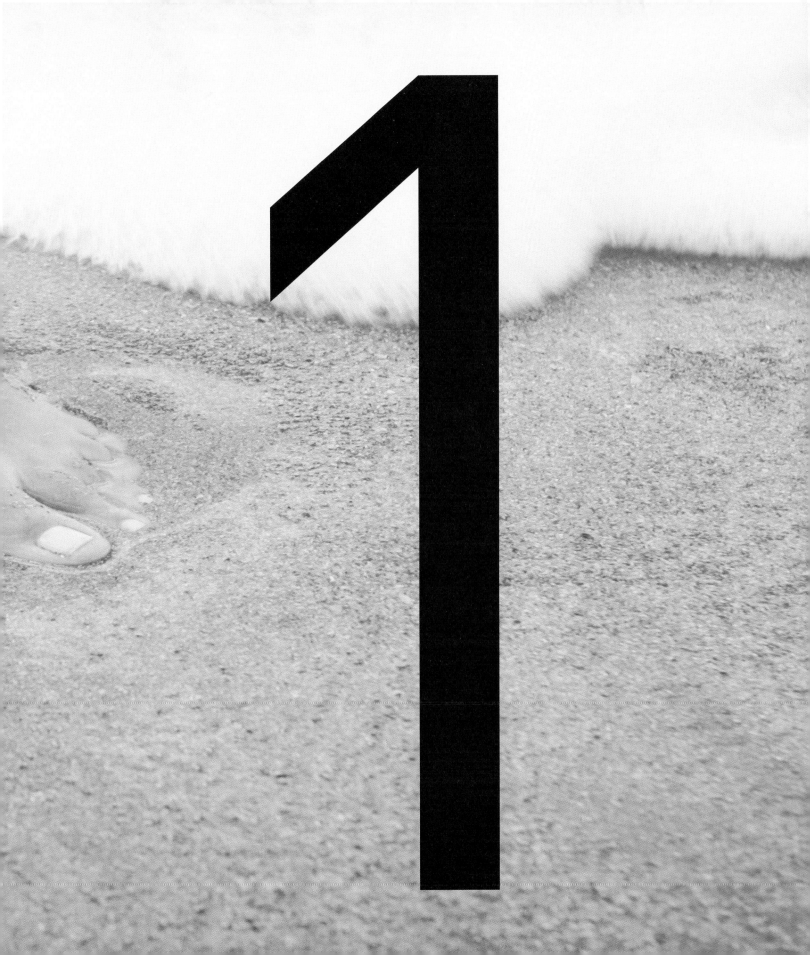

For many of us, the aging process is the primary motivator for our exploration of exercise programs. As we begin to notice the effects of aging, we become interested in yoga and other methods as a means to hang on to our youth.

With the current surge of interest in yoga and Pilates, many people are looking for an entry point into these methods that is not too intimidating or competitive. The people I have spoken to do not want to attend classes for fear of being forced to compete with others who are taut and toned, or for fear of being twisted into pretzels. They like the idea of the invisibility of T5T in that they can do it at home. Time is a factor too, as getting to and from classes takes up a lot of their valuable time. They love the prospect of being able to do good things for themselves in just 10 to 15 minutes a day.

Perhaps surprisingly, a significant number of the people attending my workshops have never done yoga. And the smaller group who practiced yoga in the past are now returning after years of aerobics and gym work. They are no longer attracted to adrenaline-induced exercise methods, and are seeking something that nurtures instead of "pumps."

The people who attend my workshops are looking for ways to change their lives. They are hungry for something to stir their passion, to help them feel "alive" again. T5T can be a step toward changing your life for the better.

T5T is for everyone who is looking for a program that is achievable, which doesn't take up too much time, which centers and calms them, and fills them with a sense of well-being. The enhanced flexibility, energy and improved breathing that come from practicing T5T can result in that longed-for sense of rejuvenation we are all seeking.

By following the T5T program we develop self-discipline in our lives, physically, mentally and spiritually. This enables us to contribute to our own empowerment but can also provide inspiration for others to achieve their human potential.

What is T5T?

T5T is a series of five yoga-like exercises and one rejuvenation breathing technique. Each exercise is performed 21 times, daily. Between each different exercise, the Energy Breathing technique is completed three times. The complete program will eventually take you between 10 to 15 minutes per day. The average is 10 minutes. Two optional breathing techniques for focusing one's awareness and achieving a deeper state of relaxation are also included.

When you begin learning T5T, you complete three repetitions of each exercise for the first week. In the second and ensuing weeks you simply add two extra repetitions, until you reach the full 21 repetitions. Throughout the program, you also carry out three repetitions of the Energy Breathing technique between each different exercise.

Increasing repetitions by just two per week allows you to progressively build up strength, as muscles take time to develop. Be prepared to take your time; it should take you around 10 weeks to achieve 21 repetitions, but you may find that you reach 21 repetitions of one posture, but remain at a lesser number of repetitions of another for several weeks. This is fine. It's much more important that you do yourself no harm. Allow your body to guide you, and you will eventually be able to do all five exercises the required 21 times each. The reason why the number of repetitions does not exceed 21 is a mystery. I have found that practicing more than 21 repetitions does not increase the energy and benefits already generated, and for some people it actually depletes them. Twenty-one repetitions seems just "right."

In the beginning you will most likely need to allow more than 10 minutes to complete your program. Remembering what to do takes time, as does building up the strength and flexibility to do the postures at a smooth, continuous pace.

If you already attend yoga or Pilates classes

If you have been doing Pilates regularly, you may have already developed strength and control of your core stability muscles. You may also have learned how to focus your mind, to control and correctly align your body, and to move with precision. These skills are equally important for T5T.

Those of you who practice yoga weekly are likely to have similarly developed strength and control. However, if the development of strong core stability muscles has not been part of your yoga regimen, you will need to allow time for these muscles to strengthen. In Part Two, I explain how these deep core stability muscles protect your spine, regardless of your level of fitness.

In either case, it is understandable that you may wish to progress through the steps at a faster rate. Be alert to changes in the energy system of your body, and possible detox effects. Pay particular attention to the Spin, as this is not part of a yoga or Pilates practice, and will therefore be new to you. You should build up the number of repetitions of the Spin gradually, stopping each time you reach a level of mild dizziness.

The Five Rites

Some of the popular yoga methods that are being taught in the West today have only been developed within the last 50 years. But regardless of the technique, all modern yoga has its roots in an ancient practice that has been in existence for more than 5,000 years.

Reminiscent in some ways of Hatha yoga postures—except the Spin, which is unique—the Five Tibetan Rites of Rejuvenation are also possibly centuries old. An indication of their age is that they are simple: just five postures. The more advanced a civilization, the more detailed and complex its systems become. Yoga originated

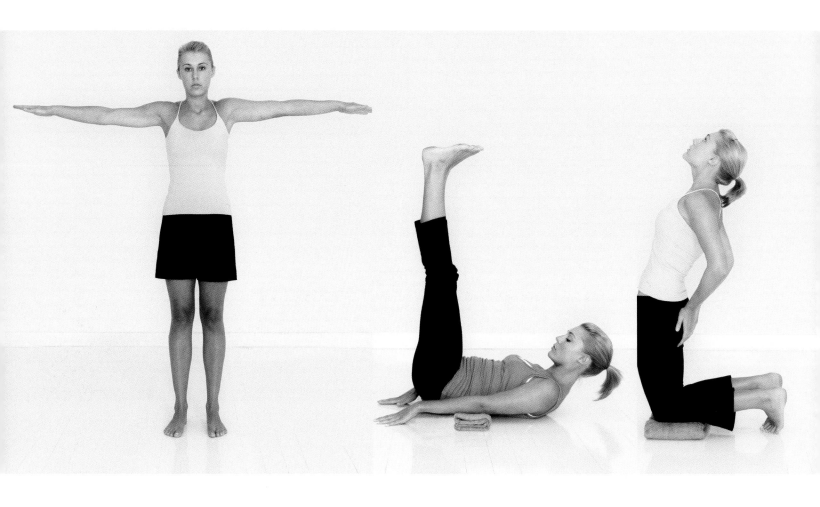

with just one meditative pose, the Lotus. Different postures were added over time to keep the spine flexible, until today there are literally thousands of them. Yet the word *asana* (a Sanskrit word referring to the various yoga postures) means "seat" or "sit in a particular position."

Hatha yoga strives to develop the physical strength and stamina necessary for the mind to remain calm and still, and for the body to remain youthful and free of disease. The Five Rites program offers the benefits of yoga, but delivers them in a much shorter amount of time. The Five Rites are also less daunting to learn than Hatha yoga, and students find it easier to maintain a constant practice.

As I outlined earlier, the Five Rites were introduced to the West by a retired British Army officer, Colonel Bradford. While stationed in India he learned of a particular monastery where the lamas were rumored to have discovered the legendary fountain of youth. The monks apparently lived to a ripe old age, without illness or any of the usual afflictions of aging.

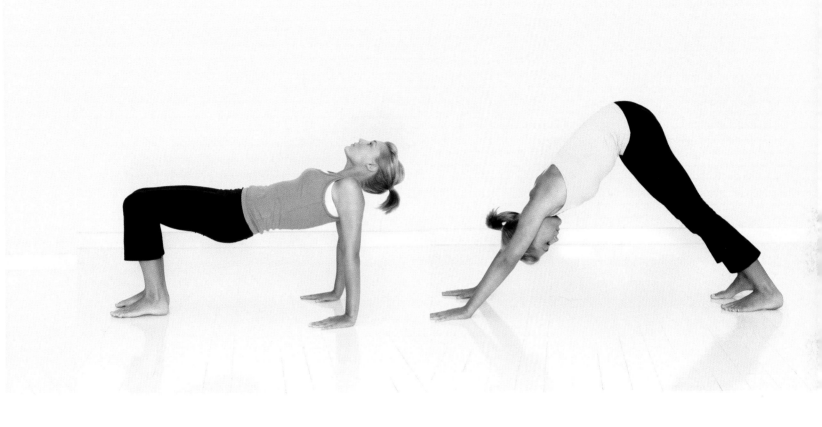

As Colonel Bradford began to age, he became obsessed with a desire to find this secret monastery in the remote Tibetan Himalayas. Before his departure he befriended the writer Peter Kelder, who would later come to chronicle Bradford's remarkable adventure.

Many years passed before a letter finally arrived from the colonel, reporting that he had achieved his goal and was shortly returning home. By this time, Peter Kelder hadn't seen Colonel Bradford in many years, and at first glimpse he didn't recognize him. Instead of an old man he saw a man years younger, whose vitality and appearance resembled how he may have looked in the prime of his life.

The colonel attributed his youthful appearance to the five yogic-like postures he had learned from the monks, which he proceeded to teach to Peter Kelder.

Peter Kelder's book on the subject, *The Eye of Revelation*, was first published in 1939. In 1985 the book was updated and republished under the title *Ancient Secret of the Fountain of Youth*. This book has sold over two million copies.

Some people believe the story; others find it too fanciful. My personal experience is that regardless of its origins or authenticity, I have taught over 700 people these same Rites and all have received the benefits Peter Kelder mentions in his books.

Quite a few people who have attempted to learn the Rites from one of Kelder's books have attended my workshops. Prior to taking my classes, they had difficulty understanding how to perform the movements, or voiced concerns about whether they were doing them correctly. Part of the problem is that the Rites are actually a dynamic, flowing series of movements. They are not static, and the original illustrations are very limited. This book moves beyond Kelder's simple presentation to include detailed instructions, a step-by-step beginner-to-advanced process and numerous supporting photographs.

In teaching the Rites, I am acutely aware that many people are simply not yet ready to achieve the original postures. They need to build up their strength first, and they also need to make necessary modifications and adaptations to suit their individual needs. Students need to learn how to protect and lengthen their spine and neck; how to keep their chest open and shoulders down; where and how to adjust the placement of their hands and feet; and how to breathe correctly. They also need to understand what *not* to do.

Most students do not know how to take a full, deep breath, or how to breathe optimally while doing the postures. These things take time to learn, and the breathing and postures are best taught in stages, leading people gradually toward their objective. A step-by-step progression is vital to successfully achieving the Five Tibetan Rites of Rejuvenation and Energy Breathing, and this comprehensive manual will help make it happen.

How does T5T work?

The connection between emotional pain and ill-health is undisputed. The Rites act on this connection by addressing all aspects of your life—physical, mental, emotional and spiritual. The T5T exercises create a profound sense of well-being by contributing to health on more than just the physical level. You will experience increased harmony and balance, with a corresponding decrease in tension, anger and negativity.

According to the Tibetan lamas, the only difference between youth and old age is the spin rate of the chakras (the body's seven major energy centers). The lamas believe that the Five Rites stimulate all seven chakras to spin rapidly at the same rate. When the spin rates are normalized, the old person becomes young again.

While I cannot prove that the lamas' assertion is true, I can absolutely verify from my observations and feedback that just about everyone who practices T5T experiences more energy, vitality and strength, an improved sense of well-being and increased personal power. Now, that sounds like feeling younger to me!

Amid the swirling, confusing, unfocused energies of the modern world, there is a light, a calm and a healing in the center of All things.
Yogi Bhajan

Life energy

The lamas believed that the aging process can be defined by the level of activity in one or all of the chakras. Ideally all the chakras should be spinning at the same rapid rate, working harmoniously together. If any one of the chakras is blocked and its natural spin is slowed, then vital life energy cannot circulate, and illness and aging set in. The chakras that are moving too slowly cause the body to deteriorate and age faster. The chakras that are spinning too quickly cause anxiety, nervousness and exhaustion. The Five Rites speed up the chakras that have slowed; bring into balance those whose spin rate is excessive; assist the body's energetic system to function normally; and coordinate their spin rates to work together harmoniously.

The T5T program harnesses and develops this highly complex system of life energy. The Chinese call this energy *Qi* (pronounced "chi"), the Japanese *Ki,* and in India it is called *prana*.

Acupuncture deals with the flow of life energy through the body, and has been successfully practiced for thousands of years—regardless of the fact that there is no precise scientific explanation to determine why the technique has positive effects. According to Traditional Chinese Medicine, a life force known as *Qi* flows through energy pathways (called meridians, or *nadis* in India) throughout the body. The correct flow of *Qi* is believed to create health; an imbalance of the flow of *Qi* creates disease. Where the energy pathway is close to the surface of the skin (known as acupuncture points), fine needles are inserted to restore balance to the flow of *Qi*.

The literal translation of *prana* is "the breath of life." The yogic concept of *prana* signifies many things: the breath, the individual and universal life force, air and strength. Although we cannot physically see this life force, and Western instruments cannot measure it, it affects every aspect of our life as it circulates throughout our body, including our thoughts and feelings as well as our physical well-being.

Chakras

Chakra is a Sanskrit word meaning "wheel" or "vortex." The chakras act like an electricity transformer, receiving and regulating life energy and transmitting it throughout the body. The Five Rites may seem deceptively simple, but they are very powerful—like flicking the energy switches in the body to ON.

Ancient Hindus distinguished seven major chakras, each one represented by a different color. There are also minor chakras in various parts of the body, including the hands and feet. The first chakra is located at the base of the spine, and the seventh chakra is on the crown of the head.

The T5T exercises stimulate the flow of life energy through the seven major chakras of the body. The chakras' energetic locations correspond with various nerve plexuses and endocrine glands, forming a bridge between our "energy" body and our physical body. Thus we can see how the lamas associate health with a free and abundant flow of energy through the chakras.

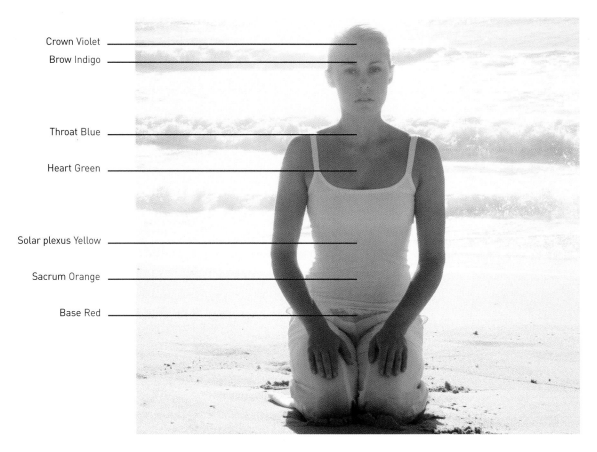

Crown Violet
Brow Indigo
Throat Blue
Heart Green
Solar plexus Yellow
Sacrum Orange
Base Red

The location and color of the chakras

Pranayama

Breathing is more than mere respiration—it is a vibrant life force that is inspired into us at birth and expired from us at death. Just as the Latin word *spiritus* means "breath of life," the bestselling author Deepak Chopra believes that "breathing is the link between the biological and spiritual elements of our nature."

The ancient masters practiced *pranayama* (breath control) to extend the breath and therefore lengthen life. They believed that we are all born with a finite number of breaths and when we have used up all those breaths, we die.

Prana, or universal life energy, can be obtained from the sun, the air, the sea, the ground, spiritual locations, from other living things and the things we eat. Yogic breathing techniques known as *pranayama* involve the movement of the breath to regulate the flow of *prana* throughout the body.

T5T combines yoga exercises with *pranayama* and natural full breathing. By connecting with the original energy that created life, you can restore your ability to heal and be revitalized.

Prana is the energy permeating the universe at all levels—physical, mental, intellectual, sexual, spiritual and cosmic energy. It is usually translated as "breath." Thus *pranayama* is an art and has techniques to make the respiratory organs move and expand intentionally, rhythmically and intensively. from *Light on Pranayama* by BKS Iyengar

Meditation and relaxation

Meditation is a technique that allows you to experience a sense of profound relaxation and increased mental awareness, enabling you to find more pleasure and meaning in your life through a deep sensation of inner harmony. Both meditation and deep relaxation are recommended for their impact on stress-related disorders, and are associated with improvements in health and productivity.

Through regular practice of T5T you will notice that your ability to concentrate and relax is enhanced. These two abilities are essential ingredients for meditation or relaxation techniques.

You may decide to incorporate a period of stillness and quietness into your daily T5T routine, and there are many techniques to help you achieve this relaxed state. T5T teaches you to focus on your breath to help still your mind. T5T's two optional breathing exercises (see Part 4, page 152) can lead you into a very deep state of relaxation, and they can also be used for meditation.

What will T5T do for me?

I have taught more than 700 people, and have received testimonials from a great many of my students. The results of practicing T5T are somewhat paradoxical, as students have told me that they have felt simultaneously relaxed and more alert; calm and more energetic; energized and focused; at peace and motivated.

Although I am wary of using testimonials to describe the benefits of practicing T5T, I genuinely believe it is possible to benefit from reading other people's firsthand experiences. Their words can motivate you, give you hope, and focus your expectations.

Common benefits of T5T

1. **Significant increase in energy**
   Rather than caffeine-like energy, this is "endurance energy." My students are often surprised by how much they can achieve in a day, compared with prior to practicing T5T. They find themselves going and going, completing tasks left undone for weeks, or even months.
   - I seem to be completing all the tasks I plan for each day.
   - My health has improved and I have the energy to appreciate my life and to help others.
   - I have more energy and motivation to get things done—I don't feel old.
   - I feel more alert in the morning.

2. **Sense of purpose restored**
   As important tasks are completed, more energy is released and extra time is created to focus on "special things." The result is a sense of feeling more in

Natural forces within us are the true healers of disease. **Hippocrates**

control of your own life. It is time to start that book, project, career change or workshop, etc., which has always been put off "until I have more time."

- I feel motivated.
- I have more balanced mental and emotional responses.
- I'm reenergized and validated in moving forward.
- I'm much calmer and better able to cope with my current health problem (cancer).
- I feel greater connectedness and groundedness.
- It has put me back in touch with my spirit.

3. **A sense of calmness**

My students feel and actually *are* less stressed. The breathing exercises help them keep calm and remain relaxed, even during stressful situations.

- I'm better able to cope at work.
- I find that I have more focus and I don't freak out when I have school exams (said by a 15-year-old).
- I am definitely more focused and committed, less stressed, my thinking is clearer and I can handle day-to-day life more easily.
- T5T is good stress relief after work.
- I have experienced reduced anxiety and anger.
- I have a feeling of calm yet also an increased sense of energy.
- I am more relaxed. I feel like a weight in my neck and shoulders has lifted.

4. **Buttons don't get pushed as easily**

My students have become less combative, moody and reactive. They feel they don't have to "try" not to react; they simply stop plugging in to the conflict, drama, negativity, etc., developing the ability to witness instead of react.

- I have more of the big picture—small stuff doesn't bother me as much.
- I don't react so quickly to things that trigger me. It puts "thinking time" between emotion and reaction.
- I am coping better with kids and work.
- My emotions are balanced.
- I am very centered and calm.

5. **Razor-sharp focus**

My students have developed significant mental clarity, as if the fog in their mind has lifted. They are able to breathe in a way that does not increase anxiety, and as a result they develop a clear and calm mind, and the ability to focus.

- It has uncluttered my brain.
- My thoughts are not so scattered.

- My concentration has improved.
- My thinking is clearer, and I am more focused on one thing at a time.

6. **Less stiff**

My students feel much more flexible, and enjoy ongoing improvement. Some no longer wake up feeling stiff, and find daily activities easier without their usual degree of stiffness.
- I find that by doing the Rites daily it seems to free my body up for the rest of the day.
- I have no aches or pains after a big day's physical work.
- My posture has improved—I feel elongated.
- Stiffness is gone.
- My muscles have an elasticity that I thought was gone, never to return.

7. **Pleasure at newfound strength and tone**

My students enjoy seeing muscles appear on their arms, stomachs, hips, legs and backs. They feel stronger in life, not just in their bodies.
- I am standing tall.
- My fitness is improved.
- I have a feeling of strength.
- I'm seeing developed muscles in my arms, calves, tummy and buttocks.

8. **Sleep improves**

People sleep better. Some of my students have found that they don't wake as much during the night. Others find falling asleep easier. Most people sleep deeper and feel more refreshed on waking.
- Finally I'm getting a better day's sleep (I work night duty).
- I find myself sleeping deeper and more restfully.
- I need less sleep.

9. **General overall improvement in health**

Some people taste, see and smell more. Others have the desire to eat healthier food, drink more water, reduce alcohol or even give up smoking. Preexisting medical conditions may improve.
- I feel more alive!
- I have lost weight and am able to maintain weight loss.
- My muscle tone has increased.
- I gave up smoking.
- My symptoms of PMS improved.
- My symptoms of menopause improved.

- I have better bowel regularity.
- My eyesight improved.
- I am experiencing improved memory, hearing and sharpening of the senses.
- I have less back pain.
- My "restless legs syndrome" has disappeared.
- T5T has alleviated my leg cramps and stiffness.
- My arthritis has improved.
- I've been able to reduce my visits to the chiropractor.
- I've been able to reduce my medication.
- I don't get the dermatitis I used to.
- T5T has provided significant relief from persistent respiratory infections such as bronchitis.
- My milk supply while breast feeding has increased.
- Everyone has noticed my youthful appearance and vigor.
- I feel a robustness in my lungs I've never felt before.
- There has been a general overall improvement in my health—I am eating better.

10. **Sense of well-being and happiness**

My students develop a youthful glow: their eyes sparkle, and their zest for life returns. Friends often ask them if they are pregnant, in love or have had cosmetic surgery!

- I feel a general feeling of well-being. I am happier.
- Friends have commented on how well I look.
- I feel more relaxed, more in control of my thoughts.
- I feel cheerful, more enthusiastic, more positive.
- I feel a zest for life, balance and joy—I feel like a new person.
- I have much more energy and stamina than I had before.
- I've had a shift in mental attitude. I feel good emotionally as well as physically.
- I'm happier and more confident—life's a buzz!

11. **Pleasure in doing T5T**

- T5T gets me going in the morning.
- It is something to look forward to.
- The thought that I can do a daily exercise routine is positive.
- Success feels good!
- The program offers me body-building strength plus energy—but requires only a very short amount of time to complete.

12. **Breathing**

When people learn T5T they are often surprised to discover how much they have been restricting their breath in a variety of situations. They also become aware of how their breathing patterns influence their stress and anxiety levels.

- T5T has given me better breathing awareness—not so shallow and more meaningful.
- My focus on breathing, and breathing deeper, has increased.
- The breathing exercise made me realize I need to do this for life.
- Using the breathing exercise to get to sleep is great!
- I have better lung capacity when walking long distances.
- I am breathing more deeply, and am very conscious of staying calm.
- The breathing exercises have been particularly helpful in centering me in a stressful situation.

Health considerations

Whenever you begin a new exercise program, there are always health considerations to take into account. The information in this section is by no means comprehensive, and you should not substitute it for the direct advice of your doctor or professional health-care provider. I suggest you take this book with you so your practitioner can accurately assess your situation. If you suffer from any of the conditions listed below, please show your physician the suggested substitutes or alternatives that are outlined for each Rite. They are specifically targeted to assist you to increase muscular strength or to improve flexibility. These alternatives can be used until such time as you are able to carry out one or several of the Rites in the classic manner.

If you feel any unusual discomfort or pain when you begin the T5T Rites, stop practicing the exercises immediately and discuss the situation with your qualified health-care provider. If you have had a previous injury, or are suffering from one at the moment, you must check with your health practitioner to ensure that T5T will not aggravate your injury. Also, if you have a history of knee, shoulder, back or neck injuries, it is always advisable to consult a qualified medical professional before attempting any of the postures.

It's particularly important to note that the T5T exercises are not intended for pregnant women, as this is not the best time for you to begin a new workout program. If you are pregnant and have already been practicing yoga or Pilates regularly, you should discuss this program with a qualified prenatal yoga or Pilates instructor, as modifications or alterations may be possible. Some of these exercises are not recommended, however, particularly in late term. Once your baby is delivered, you'll find that the exercises are an excellent way to get yourself back into shape.

You should consult your physician before commencing T5T if you have any of the following serious medical or psychological problems:

- heart valve problems
- enlarged heart
- recent heart attack
- high or low blood pressure
- cancer
- Ménière's disease
- vertigo
- multiple sclerosis
- Parkinson's disease
- seizure disorders
- mental illness.

Also consult your physician if you are taking drugs that cause dizziness, if you have had recent abdominal or chest surgery, or if you suffer from any of the following:

- hernia
- ulcers
- hyperthyroidism
- chronic fatigue syndrome
- disc disease
- fibromyalgia
- severe arthritis of the spine
- carpal tunnel syndrome
- lower back injury
- retinal or eye pressure (glaucoma).

Possible detox effects

Due to the increased elimination of impurities and wastes, and increased oxygen in your body, you may experience some minor detox effects. You could also experience some unblocking of the human energy system. Some people experience no symptoms at all, while others experience one or more of the following:

- slight headache, as if you have given up coffee or fasted for the day
- a metallic taste in the mouth
- achy joints for a day or so
- darker, stronger-smelling urine
- stronger-smelling body odor or bowel movements
- diarrhea or strong bowel movement
- initial constipation
- slight nausea
- initial fatigue as the body balances itself
- cold or flu-like symptoms that last a day
- a runny nose as sinuses clear
- a tic or involuntary muscle movement over one eye
- a mild rash or pimples
- moodiness, either a bit snappy or teary.

Consult your physician if these symptoms are severe or if they continue for more than a few days.

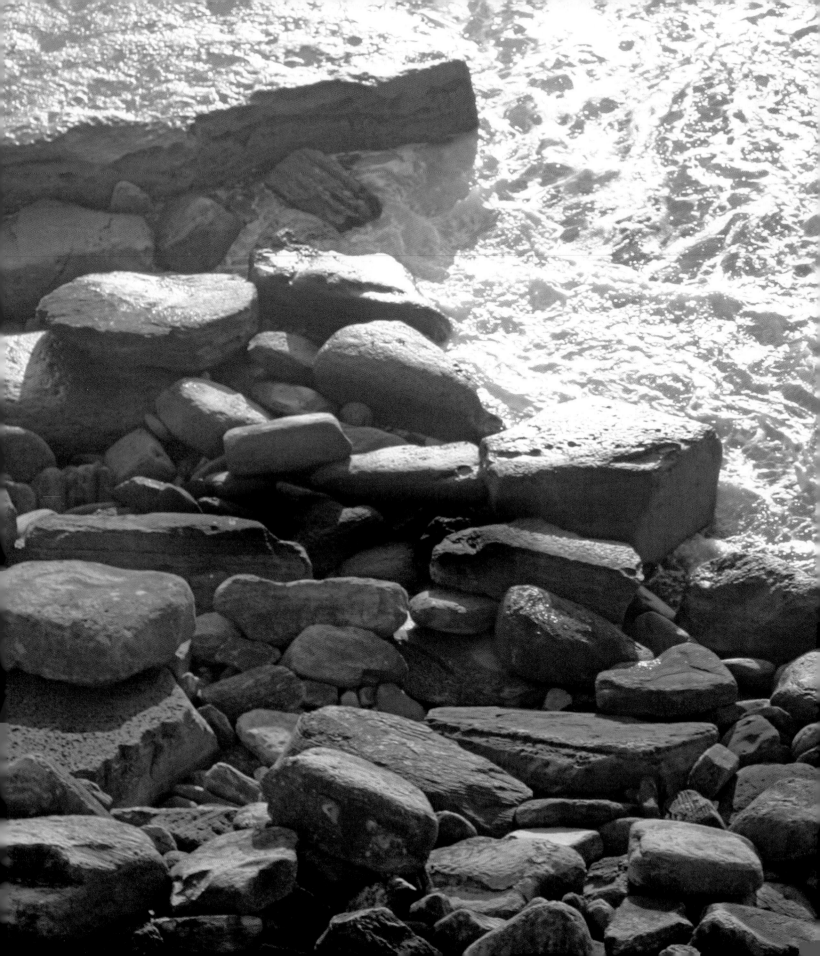

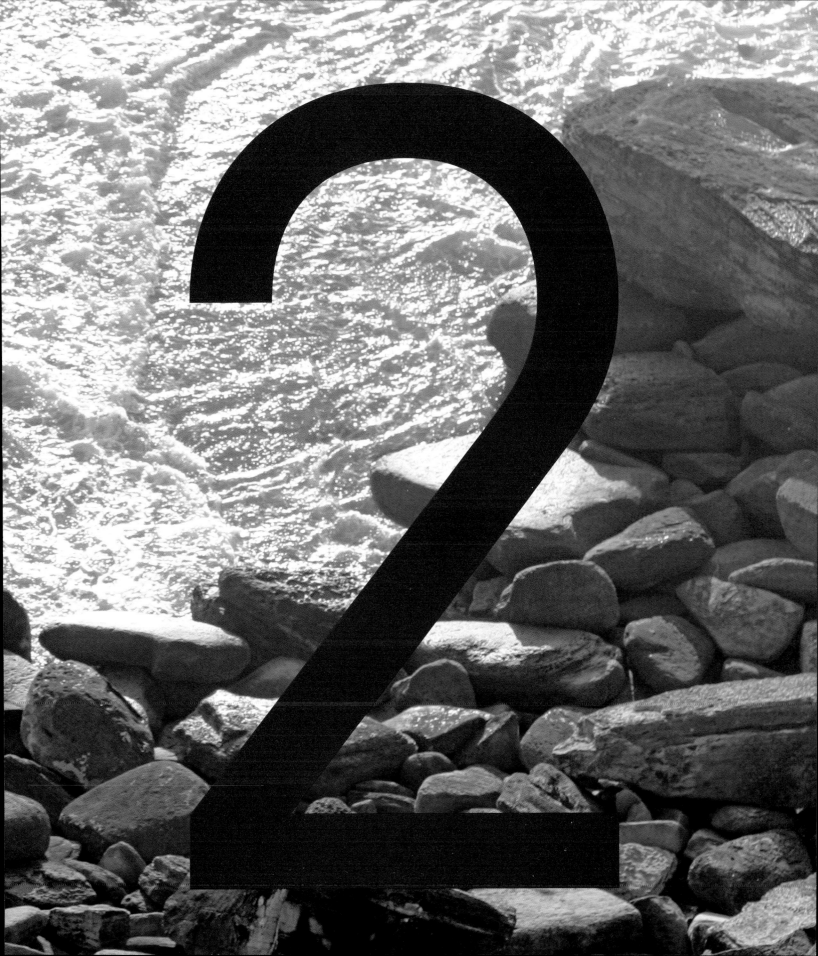

This section details the key concepts and practical skills you need to understand and develop before you start practicing T5T, readying both your mind and your body, and including aims and strategies for setting goals and achieving success. You must thoroughly understand the concepts, skills and terminology described in this chapter, and complete all the preparatory exercises that follow, before you start learning the Rites.

The first important step is to get clear on what you want to achieve from practicing T5T. This section then teaches you the important physical principles of T5T, including how to do Energy Breathing and how to activate your core stability muscles to protect your spine. A warm-up for both mind and body is also included, and the section ends with tips to keep you inspired—it's a good idea to read these tips every now and then, just to keep you on track.

You must be the change you wish to see in the world. Mahatma Gandhi

Get clear on what you want

What *do* you want out of T5T? People who end up with what they want have almost always started out with a clear idea of what that was—rather than what it wasn't! If you know what you want and understand how to achieve it, your subconscious mind will help you get there. Conversely, if you don't think your aims through before you begin, you run the risk of setting a self-sabotaging goal or outcome.

Setting your goals

Before you begin practicing T5T, it's important for you to be clear on what you want to achieve.

Get yourself a piece of paper and a pen and follow the steps from one to six below—you'll be surprised at the *real* motives this process turns up, and you may well find that you have a more expansive and longer-lasting goal than just achieving the 21 repetitions.

1. **State what you want in the positive**
    Write down what you *want*, not what you don't want.

2. **Ask yourself what you are risking if you achieve this outcome**
    Change inevitably takes us to a different place in our life. Are you prepared for this? Will you have to make some changes to your outcome to fit in with a partner or family or with work? Ask yourself what will happen if you don't achieve this outcome.

"to get rid of that persistent niggle in my back"

"to force myself to have a little 'me' time each day"

"to make me sleep better"

"to be fitter"

"to make my tummy flatter"

"to be more flexible"

"to improve my coping skills"

"to get a little perspective"

3. **Imagine you now have the outcome you wanted**
You have made it. Do you feel good about the outcome? Does it feel, look, taste, sound, smell like the outcome you wanted? Does it make sense now that you have it? Are you content with what you had to give up on the way (e.g., smoking)? If not, repeat Steps One to Three.

When your goals are clear, move on to the steps below.

4. **List the elements and resources you need to achieve your goal**
Come up with answers to the following questions: Do you have somewhere you can practice T5T? Can you fit it into your working day? What do you have to change to make that possible? Do you need a clock radio to wake you up earlier? Do you need some additional instruction?

5. **Break your goal into manageable chunks**
If you set your goals too high you will sabotage yourself. Arrange a continuous path of wins that you can achieve. Look forward along the journey of T5T and note down some stepping stones, such as: Have I practiced T5T for two weeks without missing a single day? Have I achieved this week's goal of 12 repetitions of each Rite? Charting your progress at the outset and along the way provides a measure of how much you have improved and achieved.

6. **Celebrate success**
Think of a compelling way of celebrating the successes you achieve for yourself, both along the way and when you reach your end goal. What reward will you give yourself? Think big!

By now you should be fired up and ready to move on to the physical preparation for T5T.

Breathing

If you have ever made an open fire, you know that the more oxygen a fire receives, the hotter, brighter and cleaner it burns. When a fire has plenty of oxygen it burns up all the fuel available, leaving only ash as residue. When a fire receives only limited oxygen, however, it generates more smoke, does not give off as much heat and leaves bits of fuel unburned.

An open fire can be seen as a metaphor for your breathing; the more oxygen you can breathe into your body, the more energy you will have. In addition, the more oxygen

The Lord God formed man of the dust of the ground, and breathed into his nostrils the breath of life, and man became a living soul. Genesis 2:7

your body obtains, the more waste products will be released via your respiration. In terms of elimination, respiration is as vital to your health as your bowel and urinary functions.

Over the millennia, many cultures have used breath control not only for spiritual enlightenment but also to improve health, maintain youthfulness and extend life expectancy. Modern science is confirming what the ancients believed: the way you breathe literally determines your lifespan. The total volume of air that your lungs can hold is called the "vital capacity." Now, that about says it all, doesn't it?

Deep breathers not only live longer, they live healthier and fuller lives, and are generally more relaxed and tranquil people. The way we breathe affects our nervous system. Breathing slower and deeper into the belly activates the parasympathetic nervous system associated with relaxation, and so directly impacts upon your emotions. This form of breathing helps you handle stress, improves your health and increases your energy.

Breathing too fast and shallowly into the upper chest activates the sympathetic nervous system associated with "flight or fight." This form of restrictive breathing adds to your stress and reduces your energy and vitality. People who breathe poorly suffer from anxiety, nervousness and all manner of illnesses, from heart disease to headaches, constipation to loss of vision, aches and pains to loss of memory—the list goes on.

It is important to note from the outset that the "deep breathing" referred to above is *not* the following method (best described as the Sergeant Major): stand up tall, pull your stomach in sharply and thrust your chest and spine forward; breathe in forcibly through pinched nostrils and lift your shoulders up and down. Boy! No wonder we find that so difficult and unpleasant!

True breathing is relaxed and easy; it is not the result of effort and strain as in the above example. Pushing simply causes constriction, and breathing becomes an effort. Instead of freeing the breath, the breath becomes restricted and more tension builds in your body.

With a supple belly, your diaphragm is able to move freely upward and downward in your chest. As you breathe in, your diaphragm moves downward, allowing your lungs to expand with air. As you breathe out your diaphragm rises upwards, expelling waste from your lungs.

When you breathe correctly, your whole body breathes. Like a wave, the breath flows through your being, swelling and expanding with the inhalation, and retracting and releasing with the exhalation. True breathing is when we are able to inhale fully and exhale fully, using the natural range of movement inherent in our diaphragm, belly, ribs, sides, back and chest. The depth to which you breathe and the speed of your breathing spontaneously adapt to the actual needs of the moment.

Visualization plays a significant part in maximizing the benefits of breathing deeply and slowly. Think about what you are breathing in. Perhaps it might be the air near the ocean or a waterfall. Let this beautiful oxygen- and nutrient-rich air fill every single cell in your body. As you breathe in, visualize the bountiful *prana*, the life energy you are breathing into your body. With your mind, you can direct *prana* to areas of your body that require healing or to relieve discomfort. When you breathe out, imagine the waste, toxins, tensions and worries leaving your body.

Breathing correctly

There is no single method of breathing correctly in every situation. Rather, your breathing should be able to effectively and spontaneously adjust itself in response to your activity. For example, when you are reading a book your breathing will be much slower than when you are running around the block. Your breathing also changes in response to stress, or even when you just *think* about a stressful situation.

Most people limit the amount of air they breathe; they either forget to breathe, hold their breath or breathe too much or too little. Many people pull in their stomachs, reducing the amount of air they can take in. Some people breathe so fast that they no longer experience the pause after exhalation, preventing the inhalation from arising naturally by itself. In these and many other ways, we restrict the freedom of our breath. The result is tension and stress. As Michael Grant White says, "The way you breathe can make you sick. It can also make you well!"

Don't expect your breathing to have the same pattern every day, as your breath is the first function of the body to be affected by how you feel. Whatever happens in the mind, influences the breath. Through daily awareness of your breath you can gradually reverse this process, as changing your breathing pattern can influence your mind. In other words, **to *BE* calm, *BREATHE* calm**.

How do you breathe?
Breathing rate

Current medical opinion is that 12 to 14 breaths per minute is considered "normal." Michael Grant White of Optimal Breathing at www.breathing.com, whose normal rate is 8 and resting rate is 6, believes that "normal" is not optimal, nor even healthy. He claims that unless your breathing rate is already low, you can definitely benefit from slowing down your breathing.

In teaching chronic heart failure patients (CHF) how to breathe, researchers at the University of Pavia, Italy, discovered that slowing the respiratory rate to six breaths per minute reduced shortness of breath and improved pulmonary gas exchange and exercise performance in patients with CHF. Practicing slow and deep breathing thus can be beneficial in heart failure or in other diseases. (Source: *Lancet*, 1998 May 2; 351(9112):1308-11.)

Breathing in, I calm body and mind,
Breathing out, I smile.
Dwelling in the present moment
I know this is the only moment.
Thich Nhat Hanh, Vietnamese
Buddhist monk nominated for the
Nobel Peace Prize in 1967

Before you learn the Energy Breathing technique used in T5T, complete the following test from Michael Grant White. In this exercise you count the number of complete breaths you take in one minute. When you have been practicing T5T for a few months, repeat the test and note the difference.

While sitting or lying supine, a complete breath includes one inhale and one exhale plus a pause after the exhale. Count the number of complete breaths you have in one minute. If you are unsure of the count, repeat the test two or three times, or until the number of breaths is identical (or nearly) for two sequential minutes.

Reverse breathing
Some people pull their stomachs in as they breathe in, a process that is called reverse breathing. The correct way to breathe involves a natural and effortless extension of the abdomen when we breathe in, and a flattening back of the abdomen toward the spine when we breathe out. This is called belly breathing; see page 39 for more information on this important aspect of T5T.

Chest breathing
As we grow older, we can acquire poor breathing habits and either overbreathe or underbreathe. In chest breathing the abdomen is held tense or pulled inward, preventing the diaphragm from descending fully and forcing the breath higher into the chest. It is frequently accompanied by the shoulders moving up and down.

Chest breathing is often the result of fashion's demand for a flat stomach, or it can be the result of chronic, habitual stress. Breathing in this way causes tension in the upper body because you are relying on the secondary respiratory muscles rather than on your primary respiratory muscle — the diaphragm. It also reduces your ability to breathe in or out fully. Chest breathers may compensate for the lack of oxygen by breathing more rapidly than their needs or activity demand.

Chest breathers constantly stimulate their sympathetic nervous system associated with "flight or fight," keeping themselves in a state of chronic, ongoing anxiety with associated risks to health.

Underbreathing
If you shallow breathe or hold your breath regularly, you are probably hungry for air. Perhaps you yawn or sigh a lot? Depriving yourself of oxygen by underbreathing reduces your vitality and self-empowerment. It's hard to express yourself fully when you are only "sipping" in air or if you keep running out of oxygen.

Overbreathing
Most people think that carbon dioxide is just a waste gas, but in fact it is essential for the activity of our respiratory system, heart and blood vessels. Whereas plants utilize

carbon dioxide and produce oxygen, we utilize oxygen and produce carbon dioxide. Balancing the ratio between carbon dioxide and oxygen in your body is a vital step toward achieving better health.

When you try to compensate for lack of oxygen by increasing the number of breaths you take or by breathing too fast for your actual needs, you release carbon dioxide too quickly and your body cannot use the oxygen you are inhaling. The lowered levels of carbon dioxide in your blood cause the blood vessels to constrict, thereby reducing the flow of blood and oxygen throughout your body. The result is hyperventilation, which makes us anxious and tense, and has serious long-term impacts on our health. It can also produce more immediate symptoms such as headaches, muscular tension, dizziness, breathlessness and lack of concentration.

The solution is to notice when you are breathing too fast, by carrying out the following steps:

Exercise

- First check that you are breathing through your nose, then begin to breathe slower and deeper into your abdomen.
- Relax any tension in your shoulders and focus on increasing the length of your exhalation.
- Allow yourself to experience a pause after exhalation, allowing the inhalation to arrive by itself naturally.

How to breathe while doing the Rites

While you are practicing the T5T movements, breathe in and out through your nose. This cleans and warms the air, and slows down your breathing and allows more time to focus on the mechanics of your breathing. Allow your breath to guide the exercise, breathing yourself into and out of each movement.

The natural rhythm of the breath

The natural rhythm of your breath has the following pattern: exhalation, pause, inhalation.

In T5T you focus on the exhalation, not the inhalation, as is more common. You pause after exhalation, allowing the inhalation to arise by itself.

Exhalation

Unless you breathe out fully, you cannot breathe in completely. If you extend your exhalation to its full conclusion, a deeper inhalation will occur naturally and a greater amount of oxygen will be made available to your lungs. You can never totally empty your lungs, though, as a portion of air will remain in your lungs to keep them from collapsing.

You are trying too hard if you find yourself suddenly grabbing for air. Let your exhalation lengthen naturally, without any strain. Concentrate on slowing the air leaving your body.

Long exhalations are calming. They are intuitively a time to let go and release. As you breathe out, let all your muscles relax. Feel the tension leaving your body.

Pause

The pause after exhalation is a period of natural calm and stillness, where the body's muscular and nervous systems readjust for a reversal of direction. Many people are so used to hurrying that they grab for air, leaving no time for pauses.

Let yourself relax in the pause as long as is comfortable, and then let your inhalation arise naturally.

Inhalation

The inhalation process begins with the contraction and lowering of the diaphragm. As the diaphragm descends, it displaces the soft contents of the abdomen, causing the abdomen to bulge outward. When the diaphragm relaxes on exhalation, the belly flattens.

As the diaphragm descends, the air enters the lungs from the top down. The lungs are rather like upside-down trees (the bronchial tree). As the air enters the lungs, it branches out left and right and then fans out from the center to the outside. When you exhale it does the reverse.

Monitoring your breathing is also one of the best indicators as to whether you are straining. If your breathing becomes labored, consider what your body is trying to tell you. If you are holding your breath, it is a sign that you may be pushing yourself too much. If this happens, adjust your breathing to synchronize and flow with the movement. Whatever level you are at, remember to flow with the movement and it will flow with you.

As your breathing gradually becomes longer and deeper with practice, you will be able to synchronize the timing of your breath with the duration of your movement. You will also begin to develop a sense of your breath flowing into the areas you are moving into.

T5T Energy Breathing

Energy Breathing is a vital component of the T5T exercises. Each Rite is followed by three deep "energy breaths," to help improve your stamina, boost your energy and help de-stress you.

Energy Breathing is yoga for the breath! Its purpose is to gently stretch, strengthen, open and expand all your respiratory muscles. The long, slow exhalation

Breathe deeply and gently through every cell of the body, laugh happily, and release the head of all worries and anxieties; and finally breathe in the blessing of love and hope that is flowing in the air, and you will understand the meaning of the human breath. Pundit Acharya, Indian mystic and author of *Breath, Sleep, the Heart, and Life*

is intended to calm and de-stress you as it stimulates your parasympathetic nervous system. Allowing the pause after exhalation, and then the inhalation to arise naturally, is a reminder of the need to slow your breathing. Some people have no pauses at all in their lives!—they are so busy rushing for a future event, they lose the ability to be present right now.

When you practice Energy Breathing with real awareness in the present moment it is wonderfully fulfilling and very calming. When you have mastered it, it is smooth and even and fills you up without any strain at all. You can feel the breath massage your spine and your organs as it rolls up and down your body. The exhalation is a marvelous opportunity to "let go" in the largest sense of the word; and the inhalation allows something new and fresh to come in.

These deep and fulfilling breaths are an important part of your practice in terms of vitality, mental clarity, focus and calm; they complete each posture and prepare you for the next one. Don't rush through them. Enjoy the peace that comes at the end of each breath before moving on to the next Rite.

This daily reminder of your breathing will also help you to become more aware of your day-to-day breathing pattern. You will notice when you are restricting the full potential of your breathing, and will become alert to the particular situations that trigger this response. By changing your breathing, you can adjust your reaction. How much easier would it be if you could "breathe your way" through anger, instead of suppressing it or expressing it?

Becoming aware of your breathing provides you with an opportunity for self-study. As you become more conscious of your unique breathing patterns in all circumstances, you gain more self-knowledge and awareness. It really is possible to change the way you *live* your life by the way you *breathe* your life.

The Complete Yogic Breath

T5T's Energy Breathing method is my adapted version of the well-known yogic breathing technique the Complete Yogic Breath. The first part of learning Energy Breathing is to learn to do the Complete Yogic Breath. Energy Breathing's variations include extending the exhalation, resting in the pause and allowing the inhalation to arrive by itself. I have also added affirmations, visualization and a mantra.

I call it "Energy Breathing" because it reduces fatigue, lifts your spirits, restores calm and improves your well-being. The type of energy I am referring to is not a caffeine-like instant high that exhausts quickly, but a calm, sustaining, enduring kind of energy. The former type of energy burns you out, while Energy Breathing replenishes you.

With time and practice your lungs will become more elastic and mobile. As you learn to breathe more fully and deeply you will experience a new awakening of energy and enthusiasm for life.

It's vital to practice Energy Breathing in an environment that is free from any pollutants. You will be pulling air deep into your lungs, so the fresher it is, the better. Do not use incense or expose yourself to smoke or other harmful substances, and avoid extremely cold or hot air.

Preparation

Note: The Complete Yogic Breath (or the 3-Part Breath, as it is also called) is taught differently from teacher to teacher. You may have been taught to exhale in the reverse order to that in which you inhaled. In T5T you will exhale in the same order as you inhaled—from your abdomen first, then your ribs, then your collarbones. I have tried both methods and the latter method is more popular. It more closely follows the movement of the diaphragm, which descends on inhalation and rises on exhalation. A good way of visualizing this is to imagine a bicycle pump held upside down; when you stretch it downward it fills with air and when you push it upward it pushes air outward. This analogy is similar to the action of the diaphragm.

The Complete Yogic Breath begins with a full exhalation. The ensuing inhalation is experienced first as expansion in the belly, then it rises and expands the ribs, and finally it rises and expands the upper chest. When it expands the upper chest, the collarbones and shoulders slightly rise. Breathing out is in the same manner, with the belly flattening back toward the spine. This is one complete breath. There is no pause between each stage, just a deep rhythmic movement in and out.

You will need to learn each step individually, breathing from the belly, the rib cage and the collarbones. Once learned, each step will flow into the other in one single, smooth and continuous movement. You will eventually be performing these breaths standing, lying or kneeling, according to the different instructions that follow each Rite, but it is easiest to learn each step lying down.

For this exercise it is best to wear loose clothing. You will need a scarf, sash or dressing-gown cord. The fabric must have some yield to it; a belt, for example, would not be suitable.

Begin by lying on your back on the floor. Place a blanket underneath you for comfort if needed. Place a small pillow or folded towel under your head and neck so that your chin does not tip backward or too far forward. Your throat should be soft rather than strained. Rest your arms by your sides, palms open and relaxed.

If you find this exercise hard to complete in the way described below, do not start straining to achieve it. When we learn new things it is important to remember the sequence first. With repetition the connection between your mind and body is enhanced and your body will find it easier and easier. Straining is counterproductive and only causes more tension.

Step One: Belly breathing

Belly breathing allows you to get the most air; your lungs are larger toward the bottom than at the top. A relaxed belly assists the diaphragm.

Exercise

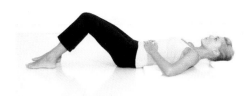

- Exhale fully before inhaling.
- When you inhale, imagine that you are blowing up a balloon. As you fill the balloon with air it expands, just like your abdomen should be doing. To help you feel the motion of your diaphragm, place your hands on your upper belly (see left). Your abdomen should expand outward as you inhale and flatten back toward your spine as you exhale.
- Relax your belly muscles; breathe in/belly out; breathe out/belly in.
- The idea is not to exaggerate the movement of your belly; in fact, the more relaxed your abdominal muscles are, the more fully your diaphragm can move, enabling more air to be drawn into the lungs. Try this exercise several times until you are confident with this concept.

Step Two: Rib breathing

Rib breathing uses the muscles of the rib cage (the intercostal muscles). By itself this is an incomplete form of breathing. During inhalation the rib cage moves upward and outward, and when you exhale it collapses, moving downward and inward.

Exercise

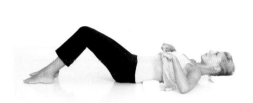

- Sit up and position your scarf or sash behind your back around the lower third of your ribs, just under your nipples. Hold the ends while you lie down again.
- When you are lying down, cross one end of the scarf over the other in front of your chest, but don't tie the ends. Hold the material in each hand (as shown at left).
- Breathe out fully and pull each end tightly.
- Breathe in, allowing your ribs to expand against the resistance of the scarf. Let the scarf slowly slip through your fingers with the movement. Provide some resistance but don't stop the movement altogether. Don't cheat by puffing your chest forward.
- Breathe out, pulling the scarf tight again. Notice how your rib cage collapses inward.
- Breathe in, expanding your ribs against the resistance of the scarf.
- Repeat this several times until you can do it easily.

Step Three: Collarbone breathing

Collarbone breathing uses the neck and shoulder muscles. By itself, this type of breathing is shallow and only partially fills the lungs. It takes the most amount of effort for the least amount of air.

Exercise

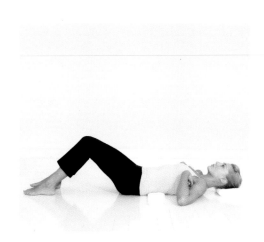

- Make loose fists with both hands and place them in or just under your armpits and apply a bit of pressure. Keep your arms upright on either side of your body. Don't let them drop beside you (see left).
- Exhale fully.
- Breathe in, allowing your upper chest to expand against the resistance of your hands, and drawing your collarbone slightly upward. The expansion felt will only be small compared to belly or rib breathing [more like a pant].
- Try this a few times without straining, feeling your collarbone and shoulders being drawn toward your head, rising with inhalation and falling with exhalation.

Step Four: Putting it all together

Now put together all the breathing techniques above in one smooth, continuous and wave-like movement—a Complete Yogic Breath. Do not pause between each step.

- Exhale fully.
- Breathe in slowly, expand your abdomen, then your rib cage, and finally your upper chest, raising the collarbone.
- Breathe out in the same manner, letting your abdomen flatten back toward your spine, your ribs retract inward, and your collarbone lower as you exhale.

Energy Breathing Exercise

In the following exercise you will learn the Energy Breathing technique used in T5T by taking the Complete Yogic Breath and adapting it slightly.

Preparation

Before you begin, it's important to understand that you should never suppress the body's natural urges. If you need to take a short breath, do so. Also, do not overdo the breathing, especially inhaling or by doing the breaths too rapidly in succession. The increased oxygen in your system can cause some people to feel a bit light-headed, dizzy, flushed or faint. If this happens, simply stop what you are doing and allow your breathing pattern to return to normal. Wait until your symptoms have subsided, then begin breathing less deeply and for a shorter period of time. You can also use up the extra oxygen by doing a few vigorous movements. Over time, your body will adapt to the new oxygen levels and these symptoms will no longer occur. Establishing a new breathing pattern takes time. Never expect immediate results.

During your T5T practice, don't rush through your three breaths. Rushing can turn an enjoyable and beneficial activity into yet another task. The breathing exercises should not be merely mechanical. Keep your awareness completely focused on your breathing as you are doing it. There are many fine points that you may miss in hurrying.

Your breathing should be slow and quiet; its volume should not change. A loud sound is a sign of straining. Aim for your breathing to be smooth, steady and even. Focus on the smoothness and evenness of your breath, gradually eliminating jerks and pauses. Relax and allow the deep calm that accompanies this deep-breathing method to settle into you.

Finally, remember that Energy Breathing should always be gentle. Never fill your lungs to their maximum capacity by blowing yourself up like a balloon, as this stiffens your body and causes strain. Proceed slowly and get to know your limits. Do not push or force your breathing in any way. You'll enjoy the experience more if you don't try too hard—Energy Breathing should not be an effort.

Step One
Remain at this level for week one of your practice.

Place your hands on your ribs just under your breastbone, with the tips of your fingers interlaced and touching in the middle (the Energy Breathing Position). You will be able to feel the expansion of your belly with your lower fingers and the expansion of your ribs with your upper fingers. As you breathe in, your fingertips will part, and as you breathe out they will come together again. This is not a big movement.

Exercise
- Place your hands in the Energy Breathing Position (see left).
- Close your eyes so you can tune in to your breathing.
- Relax your face and jaw.
- Breathe out fully to begin.
- Breathe in, expanding your abdomen, then your rib cage, and finally the upper portion of your lungs, slightly raising your collarbone.
- Breathe out slowly in the same manner, flattening your abdomen, then contracting your ribs and lowering your collarbone. Work toward gradually slowing your exhalation to about twice the length of your inhalation.
- Wait in the pause for as long as is comfortable until the new and bigger inhalation arrives naturally.
- Carry out two more extended exhalations, finishing on an inhalation.

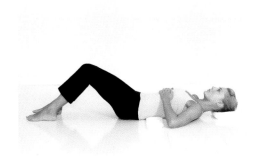

Step Two

Remain at this level for the second week of your practice.

In Step Two we are going to add a few steps:

Exercise

During the exhalation

- As you exhale, let the muscles in your neck, shoulders, chest, arms and stomach go limp, relaxing your body as you do so.
- Allow your body weight to sink deeply into your feet and into the earth below, just like a tree and its roots.
- As you breathe out, imagine you are letting go of all the tension and problems of your day. Say silently to yourself, "Let go."

During the pause

- Focus on relaxing any areas where you feel tension.

During the inhalation

- Because of the previous longer and stronger exhalation, your next inhalation should require less effort. Remember to relax your stomach and allow the new inhalation to flow in through your nose. Say silently to yourself, "This is for me."

Step Three

Commence this final level during the third week of your practice.

In Steps One and Two we focused mostly on your body. Step Three brings your mind into harmony with your body.

The following technique uses a mantra to help calm and focus your mind, so that you can enjoy every moment of your T5T practice. Then, when you have completed your daily practice, you will be able to take the energy, focus and calm you gained into your normal daily life.

A mantra is a tool to develop concentration. "So Hum" is a sacred mantra that reinforces the natural sound of breathing, and means "That I am" or "I am that." As you breathe in, say "So" to yourself and observe the natural opening and expansion you feel. As you breathe out, say "Hum" to yourself and notice how doing so seems to squeeze even the deepest air out of your lungs.

Exercise

- When you breathe in, imagine you are drawing the breath up through your feet and say "So" silently to yourself.
- When you breathe out, imagine the breath leaving through the crown of your head and say "Hum" silently to yourself.

Core stability

If you are currently practicing Pilates or any other exercise method that incorporates core stability training, there may be parts of this section that you have already studied. However, you will need to read and understand the section on how to breathe and maintain core stability during the movements on page 40.

What core stability is

All movement originates in the core of your body. Core stability works from the inside out, controlling and protecting your spine during movement by utilizing muscles that lie deep within the trunk of your body in your abdomen and back. These muscles stabilize the areas around your pelvis and spine and act like a natural corset, taking pressure off your back, pulling your abdominal muscles into place, and reducing the risk of back pain and injury by keeping your body stable and balanced.

Core stability focuses on lifting your pelvic floor and pulling your lower abdominal muscles in toward your spine. By using your abdominal muscles in this way, pulling yourself "up and in" simultaneously, you reinforce the muscles that run around and alongside your spine, creating a stable core.

Core stability training will enable you to carry out the Five Rites with control, so that you develop strength while also gaining flexibility. As you develop a strong core, you will find yourself applying this skill to other movements in your life. You'll notice that your posture is more upright, you'll look taller and slimmer, your breathing will be easier and deeper, and your movements will be more graceful.

Core muscles

Having a basic grasp of the anatomy of this area is essential to the proper practice of T5T.

The larger muscles that lie just under our skin produce movement; those lying close to the bones are stabilizing muscles that control the skeleton during movement. The trunk's stabilizing muscles are known as the core stability muscles, controlling and protecting the spine and pelvis during movement.

These deep stabilizing muscles include the pelvic floor, the transversus abdominis (the innermost layer of the abdominal muscles) and the multifidus muscles on either side of your spine. Together, these muscles completely encircle your spine from front to back like a corset, or weight belt, forming a central core. It is from this core of stability that all movements should be initiated.

The pelvic floor

The process of activating your core stability muscles begins with a voluntary contraction of your pelvic floor muscles. Think of the pelvic floor as a muscular hammock that stretches from your tailbone to your pubic bone and supports the entire contents of your abdomen. Lifting up your pelvic floor draws energy in and up the spine. The feeling is somewhat similar to when you attempt to stop the flow of urine while passing water or try to prevent yourself from passing wind.

In T5T you are going to learn how to squeeze and lift your pelvic floor muscles, resulting in a general level of stress-free, sustained support.

Exercise

- Sit comfortably in a chair with your knees slightly apart. Relax the muscles of your thighs, buttocks and abdomen.
- Without moving any other muscles of your body, try to lift your pelvic floor upward toward your rib cage.
- For women, imagine you are trying to lift up a tampon. For men, try to lift your scrotum up into your pelvis. Your testicles should lift, and your penis should withdraw a little into your abdomen.
- Relax and then try this a few more times until you are sure you are exercising the correct muscle. Try not to squeeze your buttocks or tense your thighs or abdomen.

Check that you are using only your pelvic floor muscles. In the beginning it's common to make the mistake of just clenching your buttocks and holding your breath. Other students find that they push down instead of squeezing and lifting up.

Counting out loud will remind you to breathe. Make sure you don't cross your legs or tighten your thighs or belly. Learn to isolate your pelvic floor muscles. If your stomach moves, then you are using those muscles as well.

The next time you go to the toilet to pass urine, wait until you are halfway through emptying your bladder and then try to stop the flow. Then restart it again, allowing your bladder to empty fully. Don't worry if you can only slow the stream instead of stopping it completely. If the flow speeds up, however, then you are using the wrong muscles! Only do this once a week to check your progress, as it may interfere with normal bladder function.

Multifidus

The multifidus is a collection of deep muscle bands that run up and down the spine in a diagonal direction. In some places this muscle is the size of your little finger. Its role is to stabilize the vertebrae of your back at the joint level.

When you lift up your pelvic floor and pull your lower abdominal muscles in toward your spine, a co-contraction between the pelvic floor, transversus abdominis and multifidus muscles occurs. This co-contraction enables the muscles to work in concert to provide stability to the spine.

Transversus abdominis

The innermost layer of the abdominal muscles, this broad, flat muscle runs between your pubic bone and your breastbone, wrapping around your waist and supporting your lower back. Named after the direction of its muscle fibers, the transversus abdominis muscle wraps horizontally across the abdominal wall like a corset. It is literally a natural "built-in" weight belt. It helps you breathe and protects the joints, ligaments, discs and nerves of the spine and pelvis.

You engage the transversus abdominis when you cough, laugh, sneeze or exhale forcibly.

Exercise

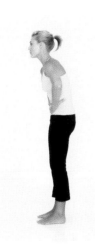

- Stand with your feet shoulder-width apart, with your knees soft and unlocked.
- Wrap your hands around your lower rib cage (see left) and cough.
- Continue to cough and feel the transversus abdominis contracting forcefully underneath your fingers.

Carry out the following "natural corset" or "tight jeans" exercise to learn how to pull your lower abdominal muscles toward your spine. You will be using this technique throughout T5T to strengthen the muscular corset around your lower torso to protect your spine. It is important to isolate the exact muscles; if your whole tummy is tensed, the stability muscles do not strengthen up as well.

Drawing the navel to the spine is often confused with sucking in the stomach. This causes you to hold your breath and negates the very effect you are trying to achieve, as it means that you are not relaxed. You need to learn to breathe normally while still maintaining the co-contraction of the pelvic floor and deep abdominal muscles.

Exercise

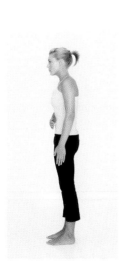

- Stand up straight with your legs hip-width apart and your knees slightly bent.
- Place one of your fingers three finger-widths beneath your belly button. Draw your stomach inward and away from your finger, toward your spine (see left). Now imagine yourself pulling up the zipper on a tight pair of jeans. Notice how you naturally lift your pelvic floor and pull your stomach in?
- Repeat the exercise until you are confident that you are isolating the correct muscles. You should be able to do this exercise without clenching your buttocks, tilting your pelvis or dropping your shoulders.

How to breathe and maintain core stability during the movements

This exercise brings together the elements of core stability—lifting your pelvic floor and the belly-to-spine technique—and coordinates them with your breath. The easiest way to do this exercise is to breathe wide into your ribs and into your back, instead of from your belly as in Energy Breathing.

Exercise

- Lie on your back, with your knees bent.
- Lift your pelvic floor and pull your lower abdominals in toward your spine.
- Breathe in for a count of two. Hold the contraction for a count of two, and without letting it relax breathe out for a count of four.
- Relax all your muscles, and breathe normally.
- Repeat the exercise a few more times until you feel confident.

Other key concepts

Here are additional key concepts you need to understand before beginning T5T.

Lengthening your spine

When practicing each of the T5T movements, including the breathing exercises, it's important to focus on lengthening your spine. Don't puff out your chest like a sergeant major; this action arches and shortens the spine. Instead, visualize yourself growing taller. Lift your sternum (breastbone) slightly, and lengthen it away from your pelvis to reduce pressure on your spine.

The lengthening of the spine allows the nerves originating from within the spinal cord to operate freely and optimally. The vertebrae are not compressed upon each other but are lengthened, giving the spine "room to breathe."

Alignment

Before each movement, check your body from head to toe to ensure that your skeleton is in the correct position to minimize tension on your joints. Neutral spine is when the three main body parts—neck, shoulders and hips—are balanced over each other and the spine has its natural curves intact. During any activity, these natural curves should be maintained, not increased. When your natural curves are properly aligned, your spinal column is in its natural neutral posture. "Neutral" alignment allows the most effective use of stabilizing and mobilizing muscles, and helps prevent back strain and pain.

In the early stages of practicing the T5T movements you will be focusing on building up strength before flexibility. Once your strength has improved, you'll be able to focus more on increasing flexibility and lengthening your spine.

Chin to chest position

In all of the T5T movements you will be asked to bring your chin toward your chest. This action stretches your neck muscles at the back and strengthens them at the front, drawing the weight of your head forward to decrease neck tension. Your head is a heavy object, and the chin to chest position works with gravity to hold it in the safest position for your neck and back. The movement also affects the deep abdominal muscles.

Exercise

- Rotate your head downward from your jawbone. As you tip your chin down, the rotation should be in the jaw joint, allowing your head to come forward above the breastbone (see left). Do not pull your chin in so far that you strain the front of your throat.

Some students jut their chin out before moving it toward their chest. This creates strain and shortens the neck muscles. The movement should be more like how a turkey pulls its head in instead of like a swan.

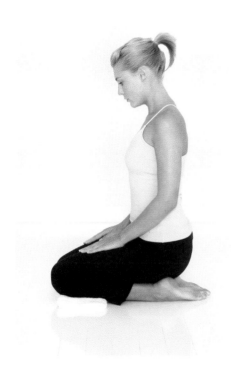

Correct shoulder position

It is very common for people to habitually hunch their shoulders toward their ears. Other bad habits are holding one shoulder higher than the other or holding your head in a forward position. Keep your head balanced evenly between your shoulders. Keep your shoulders back and down. Imagine there is a string attached to the crown of your head, pulling you upward to the ceiling. This action lengthens your neck and helps you maintain a correct head, shoulder and spine alignment.

In T5T you will learn not to elevate your shoulders during any exercise. The trick is to keep your shoulders back and down, not rolled forward and hunched upward. An effective tip is to visualize trying to place your armpits over your hipbones, but without shrinking your spine.

Preparing to begin the T5T Rites

You are now almost ready to begin the T5T Rites. Before you begin, however, it's important to prepare your mind and your body. You need to become "present in your body" before beginning to learn the movements, and the best way to achieve this is through focused relaxation. The following "Be Here Now Breath" will help you relax physically, preventing predominantly used muscles from continuing to overwork. It will also help to calm the noisy chatter of your mind. The warmup exercises that follow it stretch and ready your body for action.

The Be Here Now breathing technique

This technique is optional in T5T. The best time to use it is when your mind is pre-occupied with other things. If you feel scattered and "not present" when you do T5T, you may not be aware of when you are straining your body. The Be Here Now breathing technique helps combat the self-defeating and stress-inducing habit of rushing, and will prevent your practice from becoming just another task to be completed.

One minute is usually sufficient, but this technique can be extended for as long a period as you desire, and can be used for meditation. Several of my clients prefer to call this technique the One Minute Meditation, and use it frequently at stressful moments during their normal life.

Exercise

- Sit in a comfortable position or lie on the floor with your knees bent. Rest your hands by your sides so as not to restrict your breathing. Close your eyes.
- Exhale fully.
- Breathe in through your nose, taking a slow, deep diaphragmatic breath, and then exhale slowly through your nose.
- Continuing to breathe, mentally scan your body from your toes to the top of your head, consciously relaxing your muscles deeply as you do so. Pay special attention to your jaw and your hands, areas that typically hold lots of tension due to clenching.
- Become aware of your breathing.
- On your next exhalation, say silently to yourself "Breathing out." *Experience* yourself breathing out.
- As you pause, say silently to yourself "Pause." *Experience* yourself pausing.
- As you breathe in, say silently to yourself "Breathing in." *Experience* yourself breathing in.
- Continue in this manner, saying your breathing rhythm silently to yourself while you experience your breathing:
  Breathing out
  Pause
  Breathing in
  Breathing out . . .
- Breathe easily and naturally in this manner for one to two minutes or until you feel calm and centered.
- If you find your mind wandering, don't worry; just bring your awareness back to experiencing your breathing rhythm and saying each step silently to yourself.
- When you are ready, open your eyes and allow your awareness to come back into the room.

Warm-up exercises

These five warmup exercises focus on improving blood circulation throughout your whole body, releasing tension, removing stagnation in your muscles and stimulating the circulation of *prana*. Additional warm-ups are provided before the leg raise and the kneeling backbend to specifically target the muscle groups that are about to be used. They are designed to release tension and prepare the body for movement.

It is important that you carry out *all* the exercises below when you are learning T5T. Once your body is strong and flexible and you have developed excellent day-to-day body–mind awareness, you can include the exercises that you find beneficial and eliminate others if you wish. For example, if your body is already warmed up from a walk, you may prefer to do the stretching exercises and eliminate the shaking and patting. (Note: the swinging, shoulder rolls and neck stretch are always recommended.)

The best way of determining the appropriate type of warm-up is to scan your body for tension before you begin the Rites. You can then pat or shake into specific areas to release tension.

Exercises

Shaking

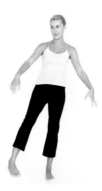

- Start by gently shaking your hands, then your arms.
- While still shaking, slowly lift your arms up over your head and then down again. As your hands and arms come downward, let the gentle shaking motion spread to your upper body, neck, shoulders and chest.
- Continue shaking all the way down your body, until your hips are shaking side to side. Your whole body will now be shaking.
- Continue that movement for a few minutes and then raise each leg in turn, shaking the whole leg, foot and ankles. Pause briefly to feel any changes.

Patting and Small Fists

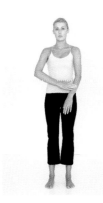
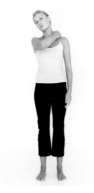

- Begin by gently patting your arms, from your wrists up to your shoulders and then up to and behind your neck.
- Spread your fingers so you can pat areas of your upper back that you cannot reach otherwise.
- Make your hands into small fists and, using the opposite arm, gently tap all around the stiff muscles around your neck, upper back and shoulders.
- Continue to use your small fists to tap across your chest, sternum and down your sides, stimulating the area around your lungs, stomach, hips, buttocks. Then up either side of your spine and down each leg.

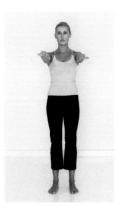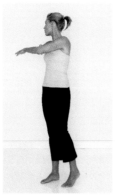

Swinging

- Stand with your feet about hip-width apart.
- With your palms facing downward, raise your arms straight up in front of you at shoulder width and shoulder height.
- Start to swing to the right by lifting your left heel off the ground and gently swinging your right arm straight behind you and your left arm across your chest. Keep both arms in line with each other.
- Now swing to the left, lifting your right heel off the floor and bringing your left arm straight behind you. Allow your head and eyes to turn with the movement.
- Without effort, allow your swing to gradually widen and continue this side-to-side swinging movement until you feel relaxed.

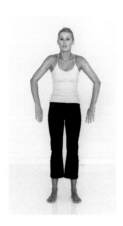

Shoulder Rolls

- Stand up straight, with your arms hanging loosely by your sides.
- Rotate your shoulders by making little circles with them in a backward direction three times.
- Come back to the middle and then rotate your shoulders in a forward direction three times.

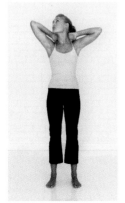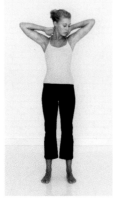

Neck Stretch

- Interlace your fingers behind your head just under the bony part of your skull.
- Slowly and gently, make circles with your head in a clockwise direction, and then in a counterclockwise direction. (Make certain that you do not push the head forward or backward—use the hands as a guide only.) Let your eyes follow the movement. Breathe in as your head rotates upward and breathe out as your head rotates downward.

You should now be nicely loosened up and ready to move on to the first Rite: the Spin. Refer to the following three important pages as needed during your practice.

Tips to keep you on track

- T5T is an activity that you can potentially carry out for the rest of your life. It works on your body, your energy system and your mind.

- Your daily T5T practice takes just 10 to 15 minutes per day.

- If you practice T5T for 90 days, you won't have to motivate yourself, as the benefits will make you want to continue to do it. You will have established a pattern as firmly entrenched as cleaning your teeth, plus you will have begun to see benefits from your daily practice of T5T. Never break the pattern of doing T5T; if you have to miss a day, due to illness, travel or work commitment, cut back your repetitions to just three or five of each or just do what you can. If you start the Spin, chances are you will continue with the rest of the Rites.

- Morning is the **best time to do T5T,** as the benefits you gain from your practice carry over into the rest of your day. Research has also shown that people who exercise in the morning are more likely to maintain their exercise regimen.

- Use visualization to enlist the power of your mind. Visualization works. Visualize yourself moving through the postures gracefully and effortlessly, like in a dance. See yourself breathing freely and in harmony with the flow of the movements. Notice how your body feels strong, supple and youthful. Notice how calm you feel and how clear your mind is. Then see yourself in your normal day-to-day life, moving with confidence and trust in your new body.

- Do the exercises in your head first, before you do them physically. When you "see" the movement first, you'll find your nervous system will work out the best way to move your muscles.

- Have you noticed how you hold your breath when you are intensely focused on something? Your eyes are most likely to be affected too, as they narrow and tense with increased focus. However, when you are in the present moment, breathing slowly and deeply, your eyes naturally "soften." With "soft" eyes you can take in all the peripheral events you might be missing by being overly focused. Try doing your T5T practice with soft eyes. You will find it's a profound experience that you will want to replicate in other areas of your life.

- Watch what your face is doing as you practice. Are you screwing up your facial muscles, squinting your eyes or clenching your jaw? If you are, chances are you are straining. Try smiling slightly. Smiling while you are practicing takes the seriousness away, and you are far more likely to enjoy yourself.

- Don't fight with your body. Simply proceed at your own pace, which will be dictated by your individual level of flexibility and strength.

- Move your body smoothly and slowly into each movement. Control your movements. Aim for muscle control without tension. Listen to what your body is communicating to you. This is the best way to enhance your awareness of your body's limitations and to enjoy its developing strength and flexibility. Calmly focus on your breath as it flows in and out with the movements.

- Smooth and controlled movements are far more effective and less stressful on your joints. Jerky movements and wild, uncontrolled movements are signs of "cheating" your way into the posture. Such lack of control also means that you are using the momentum of the movement instead of your muscles. You won't develop as much strength, flexibility or coordination in this way, and you place yourself at greater risk of injury.

- Enjoy what you are doing, and don't be afraid to adapt the postures to suit your ability. If you can't straighten your arms and legs, it's okay to slightly bend them—it's far better to bend than to try to force yourself into the full posture.

- If you are feeling pain, stop! Don't continue with the movement, hoping that the pain will go away. Take time to adjust your movements so you won't feel that discomfort again.

- Beginners often experience involuntary trembles in certain positions. This is a normal response, indicating that your muscles are adjusting to a new demand. If the trembling gets very strong, ease back or stop.

- Don't "push" past the wisdom of your body. You can only do what your body will allow you to do, and that varies from day to day. Your body never lies, and if you learn to listen to it you will develop the powerful ability to remain focused in the present moment. This ability will affect not just your T5T practice but your entire life, enabling you to be much more effective as well as reducing your stress levels. It will literally change your life if you let it.

- Be careful not to become fixated on achieving the full 21 repetitions. You'll miss the all-important journey. If you find yourself rushing, you are already in the future and not here now. If you are not in the present moment, you run the risk of strain and injury and, worst of all, you turn a potentially beautiful daily dose of self-care into just another task to be achieved.

- The simple movements in T5T contain many smaller movements, which you will need to concentrate on initially. After a while they will become second nature. If you find yourself rushing or feeling bored, this is a sign that you are "not in your body" and therefore not in the present moment. When you breathe quickly and erratically, your mind becomes scattered and wandering; if you control your breathing, you can control your mind. Take deep, rhythmic breaths to exercise your body and relax your mind. When your mind is focused and calm, your daily T5T practice is so much more pleasurable.

- Once you have felt the benefits of T5T, your motivation may waver and you might start missing a day here and there. You might start to practice the Rites later and later in the day; you might rush through them; or you might make cups of tea or put the washing on between each Rite, etc. Watch out for this.

- If you were a procrastinator before doing T5T, chances are you still will be! Everyone has this potential to some degree. The change will be that you will recognize this pattern, and will be able to take steps to prevent the usual broken agreements with yourself from taking place. This is vitally important, since every time you break a promise to yourself, it weakens your will.

- Adhering to the discipline of practicing T5T every day will make you feel more powerful, focused and energetic. I call the surge of endurance and energy and the sense of purpose that come with the daily practice of T5T "the Force." Sometimes the Force is so subtle that you don't really notice it until you review the changes that have occurred. But when you feel the Force, use it!

- If you have a calendar it is a very good idea to put a large check mark next to each day you do your T5T practice. You can't ignore a blank date box!

- A diary is useful for the same purpose, and is great for recording how many repetitions of each posture you carry out. You may find that you proceed more rapidly with some postures than others. A record helps you keep track of where you are up to in the program and what you have achieved. It is a good idea to also include observations about your physical state and state of mind. By the time you are performing 21 repetitions, in about 10 weeks' time, you will be a different person, and will have forgotten the old you; keeping track of your changes and comparing them to your goals will remind you just how much you have achieved.

- It's a good idea to learn T5T with a friend, partner or relative. You can motivate each other by telephone, no matter the distance.

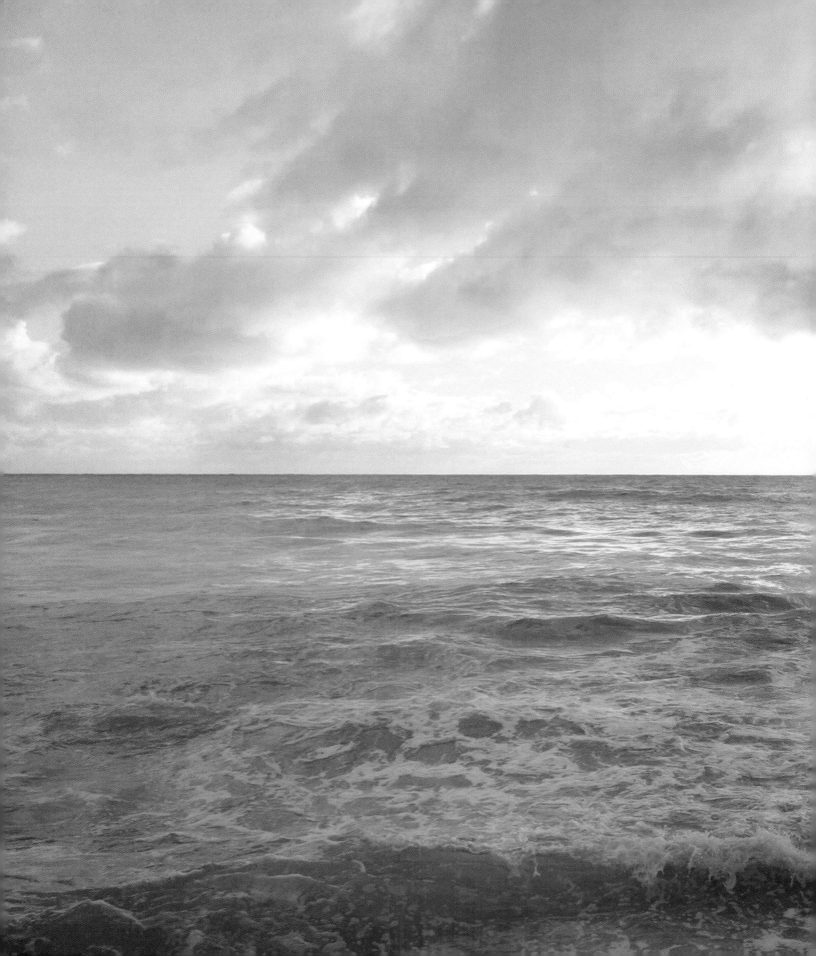

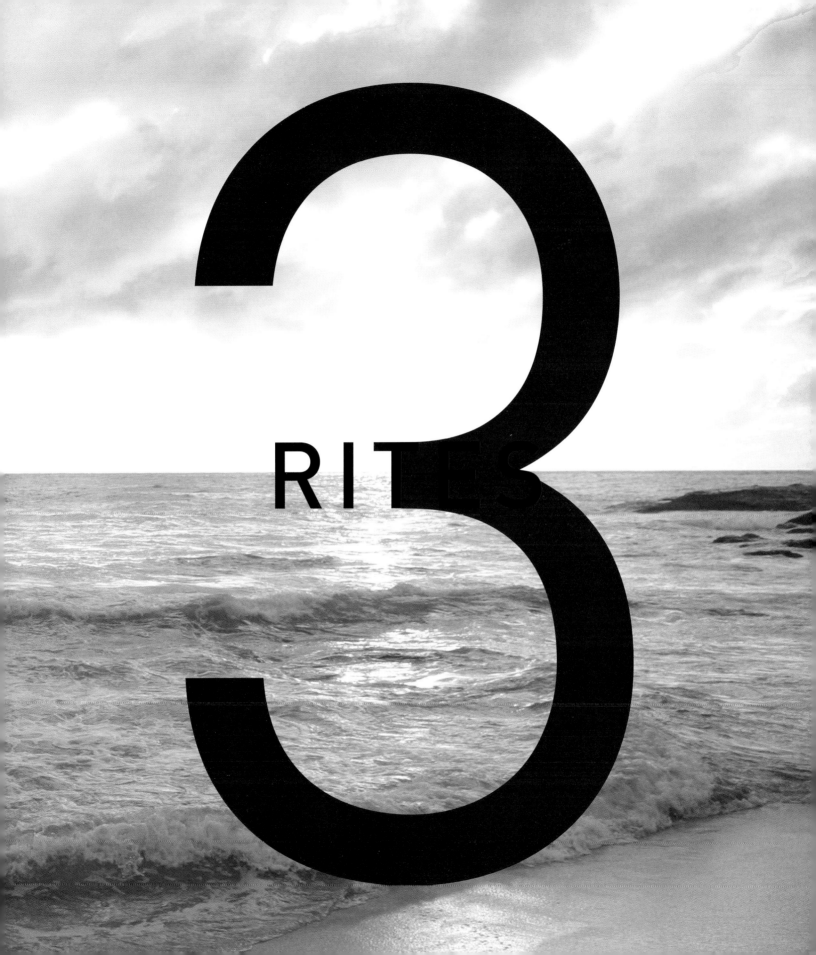

3

RITES

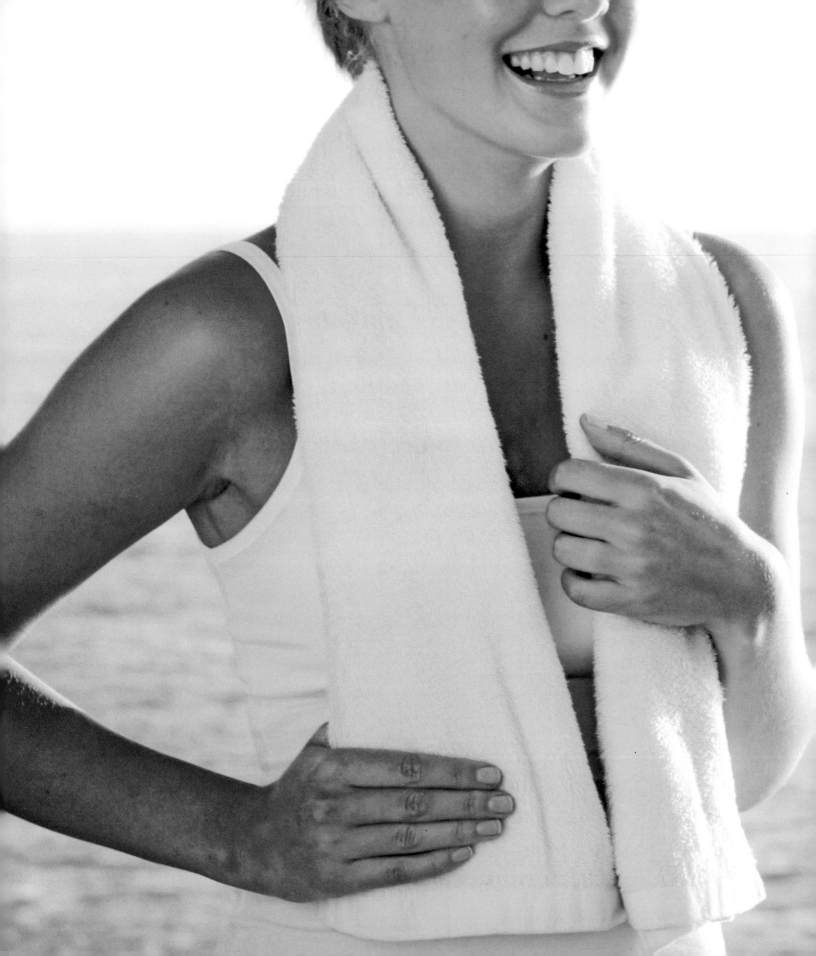

The Rites are learned progressively. In each case you begin with the basic steps or movements, learning which muscles to use and then strengthening those muscles. When you have mastered the basic steps, you are ready to move on to more advanced levels. The aim is to gradually work up to 21 repetitions of each Rite, beginning with three repetitions per day for the first week, then increasing by just two repetitions per week (see the chart on the following page for a summary of the weekly program). When you are performing 21 repetitions, T5T is yours forever and you can take your 10-minute program for health, energy and vitality with you wherever you go.

Many people claim that the best thing about the Five Rites is that you don't have to do them perfectly to gain great benefits. In each case I have supplied alternatives or adaptations that can be used in the learning process or if you are unable, for whatever reason, to do the classic version.

The other popular feature of the Five Rites is that you can do them almost anywhere at any time. With the exception of a small towel for the Leg Raise, no equipment is necessary—although you can put down a towel or yoga mat for the Rites that require you to kneel or lie on the ground, if desired.

Remember to listen to your body and its day-to-day needs in preference to any suggested program development. Do only what you can do with comfort and ease. Stay within your own limitations until you are ready to progress.

The Five Elements

At the time of the development of the Five Tibetan Rites of Rejuvenation, the ancients believed that their world was composed of Five Elements; water, earth, air, fire and spirit (energy). In psychology, the Five Elements are used to personify different human traits, such as the personality types categorized by Carl Jung (feeling, sensing, intuiting and thinking) and those associated with the astrological signs of the zodiac. I experimented with the concept of assigning an element to each of the Rites, and found the results to be amazing.

In each case, the physical movement of the Rite was a metaphor for what we were trying to achieve mentally—awareness in a different aspect of life. For example, the Spin takes the element energy, and the vortex that the movements create allows you to replenish your body from the larger energy all around us. The Tabletop takes the element earth, and its movements focus on stability, foundation and balance, giving us a solid base from which to form new ideas.

In holistic exercise it can sometimes be hard to marry the physical state with the mental state, and having a metaphor helps people enormously to align the two, and to present a clear picture of what they are working toward.

The introduction to each Rite begins with the element to which it relates and then uses this framework to tell the spiritual story of the Rite. Many people find it helpful to use affirmations during their practice of T5T, so each Rite is accompanied by an affirmation that you can say silently to yourself to focus your mind on these concepts as you perform the Rite.

Week No.	To Learn	Already learned—in sequence	Repetitions	Page
1	Step 1: Spin Step 1: Energy Breathing Step 1: Leg Raise Step 1: Kneeling Backbend Steps 1–3: Tabletop Steps 1–3: Pendulum		3 x each Rite followed by 3 Energy Breaths	62,63 35 78,79 106,107 122–127 144,145
2	Step 2: Spin Step 2: Energy Breathing Step 2: Leg Raise Step 2: Kneeling Backbend	Step 1: Spin Step 1: Energy Breathing Step 1: Leg Raise Step 1: Kneeling Backbend Tabletop Pendulum	5 x each Rite followed by 3 Energy Breaths	64,65 36 80,81 108,109
3	Step 3: Leg Raise Step 3: Energy Breathing	Spin Step 2: Leg Raise Step 2: Energy Breathing Kneeling Backbend Tabletop Pendulum	7 x each Rite followed by 3 Energy Breaths	36 82,83
4	Step 4: Leg Raise	Spin Step 3: Energy Breathing Step 3: Leg Raise Kneeling Backbend Tabletop Pendulum	9 x each Rite followed by 3 Energy Breaths	84,85
5	Step 5: Leg Raise	Spin Energy Breathing Step 4: Leg Raise Kneeling Backbend Tabletop Pendulum	11 x each Rite followed by 3 Energy Breaths	86,87
6	Step 6: Leg Raise	Spin Energy Breathing Step 5: Leg Raise Kneeling Backbend Tabletop Pendulum	13 x each Rite followed by 3 Energy Breaths	88
7	Step 7: Leg Raise	Spin Energy Breathing Step 6: Leg Raise Kneeling Backbend Tabletop Pendulum	15 x each Rite followed by 3 Energy Breaths	89
8	Step 8: Leg Raise	Spin Energy Breathing Step 7: Leg Raise Kneeling Backbend Tabletop Pendulum	17 x each Rite followed by 3 Energy Breaths	90, 91
9	Step 9: Leg Raise	Spin Energy Breathing Step 8: Leg Raise Kneeling Backbend Tabletop Pendulum	19 x each Rite followed by 3 Energy Breaths	92
10	Step 10: Leg Raise	Spin Energy Breathing Step 9: Leg Raise Kneeling Backbend Tabletop Pendulum	21 x each Rite followed by 3 Energy Breaths WELL DONE!	93

ENERGY

life force (prana, Qi), energy, spirit,
fountain of eternal youth

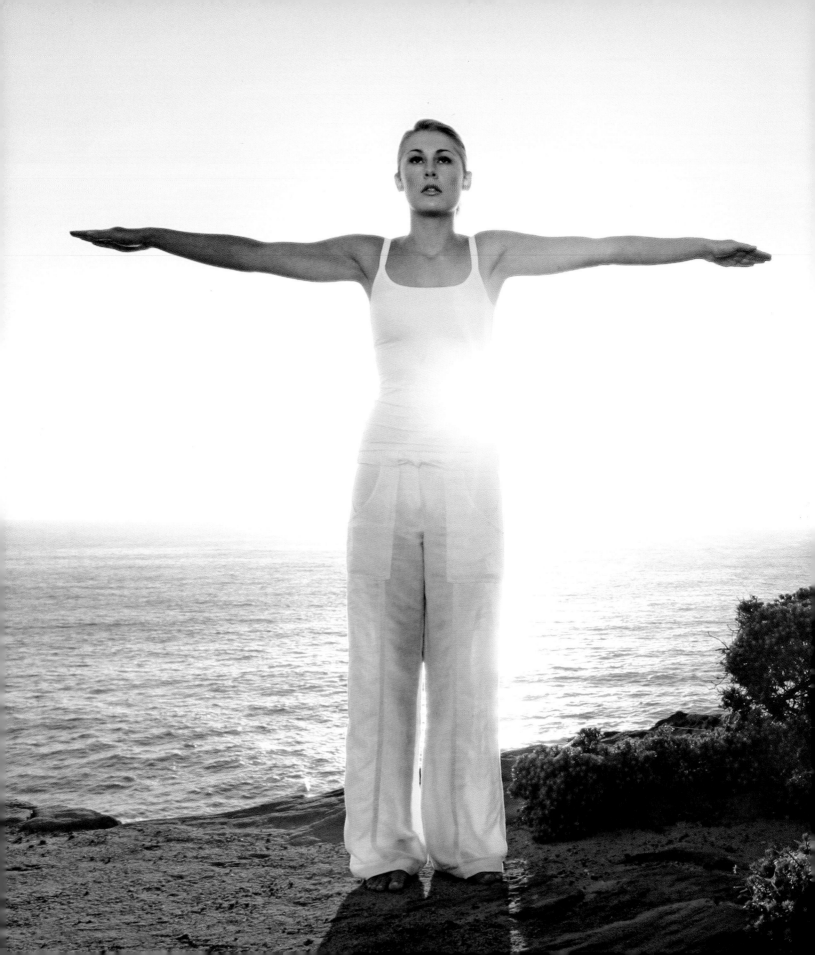

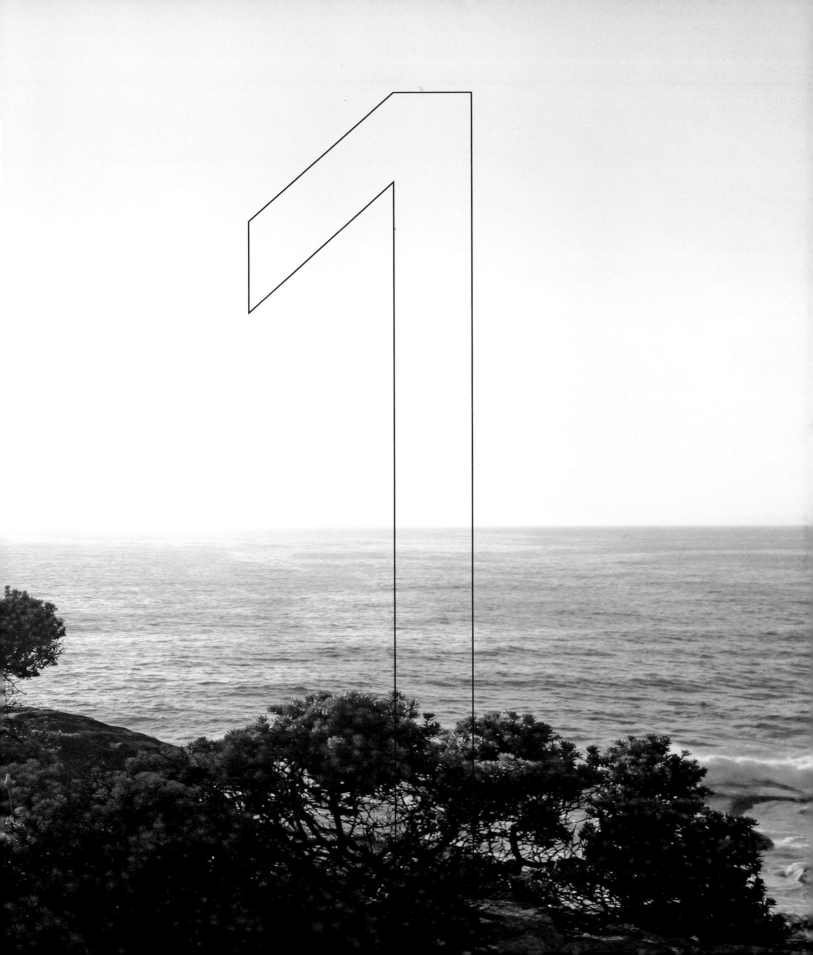

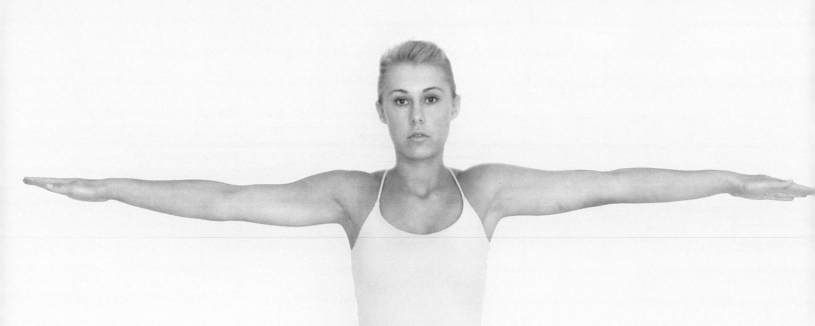

1ST RITE
THE SPIN

ENERGY The Spin represents the need to refresh, replenish and energize your body and mind. When you practice this pose, you stimulate your chakras into action, harmonizing the flow of essential life-energy throughout your body. In places where your energy levels have been depleted, vital life force (*prana*) can now enter to revitalize and recharge your body.

This "spark of life" is capable of entering every single cell in your body and into your life. Work with this extra energy by being aware of how it is energizing every area of your life. Learn to use this energy for your own transformation.

Affirmation: "I am full of energy."

INTRODUCTION

A secret turning in us makes the universe turn. Head unaware of feet, and feet head. Neither cares. They keep turning. Rumi

There is no object or being that does not revolve. From the furthest galaxy to the tiniest cell, through the revolving of the neutrons, protons and electrons of the atoms that form our basic structure, everything takes part in this revolving.

You can see evidence of spinning everywhere; even our own earth spins around the sun. When viewed from space, the large, swirling cloud formations of hurricanes, for example, are similar in shape to the swirling galaxies of other universes. Your own body contains numerous spirals, from your DNA to the unique swirls on the tips of your fingers.

The vortex formation is integral to the universe. It's a constant that recurs throughout all life. It is a revolving whirlpool of energy whose rotational power focuses and channels energy from a much more powerful source. The ancients taught that the universe is full of spinning vortexes through which the energy of the universe enters and vitalizes your body and all other things.

Ancient cultures also believed that the human body contains energy vortexes and pathways. Indian culture has kept this concept alive from ancient times until today. Indians and ancient cultures see the body as containing seven main energy vortexes, which they call *chakras,* the Sanskrit word for "wheel." They believe that these "wheels," arranged vertically from the base of the spine to the top of the head, are sites where you can receive, absorb and distribute life energies (see Part One, Life Energy, page 13).

The Tibetan lamas who developed and practiced the Rites emphasized the link between good health and the balanced and even spinning of these chakras. Their teaching, which is centuries old, explains that the Rites are a simple but powerful way to stimulate the chakras to perform and function in maximum potential and harmony.

The First Rite, the Spin, is a perfect warm-up and alignment for all the chakras of your body. Once you have mastered this Rite, you will find it a joyous experience. With your arms spread out wide beside you, you turn from left to right in a clockwise direction. As you speed up, you feel the wind on your arms and face, your body poised in perfect balance.

Those who spin

It would be natural to assume a link between the origins of the First Rite and the whirling dervishes, founded by the great philosopher and writer Rumi in the late 1200s. However, there is no evidence to support this connection. Although they both involve spinning, the First Rite and the Sema (the dance of the whirling dervish) have different purposes and vary significantly in technique.

The Sema is part of a sacred ceremony in which the dervishes spin to induce a feeling of soaring, ecstasy and mystical flight. The spinning represents the earth revolving on its axis around the sun, and creates a hypnotic and relaxing effect that opens the dervish's body to receive the energy of God. *Dervish* literally means

. . . The sky is round, and I have heard the earth is round like a ball, and so are all the stars. The wind in its greatest power whirls. Birds make their nest in circles, for theirs is the same religion as ours. The sun comes forth and goes down again in a circle. The moon does the same, and both are round. Even the seasons form a great circle in their changing, and always come back again to where they were. The life of man is a circle from childhood to childhood, and so it is in everything where power moves . . .
Black Elk, Sioux holy man

"doorway," providing an entrance from this material world to the spiritual, heavenly world. They see themselves as the conduit of God's power, and do not try to hold on to or direct that power.

During the Sema the dervishes may spin hundreds of times. The Tibetan monks, on the other hand, would only spin a sufficient number of times (21) to stimulate the chakra vortexes into action. They believed that spinning to excess (as the dervishes do) overstimulates the vortexes, causing exhaustion.

The dervishes place their right palm upward to receive the power of the heavens, and turn their left palm downward to direct this energy into the earth. In the Tibetan First Rite, however, both palms face downward toward the ground.

Despite the inherent differences in these practices, it does seem reasonable to think that there may be some universal significance in terms of the connection between spinning and energy generation and dispersal, and that there may be an even older root from which spinning springs. For example, yogis are also known to spin spontaneously when experiencing certain high levels of energy.

We can only speculate about the true origins of the Spin, yet spinning is so natural it almost certainly evolved from the careful observation of natural laws.

Direction of the Spin

When you practice the First Rite, you spin in one direction only—clockwise. Just as water spirals down the sink in apparently different directions, some people believe that we should adjust the direction of our spin in accordance with the Coriolis Effect, which is created by the rotation of the Earth. If this were the case, we should spin counterclockwise in the Northern Hemisphere and clockwise in the Southern Hemisphere. But what would we do on the equator?

In actuality, the measurable effect of this scientific phenomenon on the normal water spiraling down your sink is a myth—unless your sink is the size of a small ocean. The rotation of the Earth, and thereby the Coriolis force, is only one full rotation per day—extremely minor. (The direction of water draining is determined by earlier rotation, i.e., how the water comes out of the tap or pipes, or how it is subsequently disturbed.) The degree of Coriolis Effect on a spinning human being would therefore be negligible and impossible to gauge accurately.

The lamas instructed us to spin clockwise, but their reason for doing so has unfortunately been lost over the hundreds of years of the Rites' existence.

Interestingly, a dance teacher who attended my class told me that children are initially taught to spin clockwise. Apparently they find it easier. She said it is well known among dance teachers that if you want to calm children down, you get them to spin counterclockwise. To energize them, you get them to spin clockwise!

This energizing effect is exactly what most people find they experience when they spin.

Barbara Anne Brennan, ex–NASA research scientist and noted authority on the human energy field, says in her book, *Hands of Light,* that a clockwise spin of the chakras draws energy from the universe and a counterclockwise spin causes energy to flow out from the body, interfering with metabolism.

Benefits

The monks believed that spinning creates a vortex that aids the upward flow of vital life energy through all the chakras, helping to revitalize, stimulate and harmonize their spin rates. The Spin speeds up all the chakras and stimulates them into action.

Spinning creates movement that distributes energizing *prana* or *Qi* throughout your entire body. Where there is movement, there is life; where there is no movement, there is stagnation and eventually death.

Spinning enhances circulation and stimulates your nervous and lymphatic systems. It helps your balance and improves your coordination. As you hold your arms outspread in the Spin, your arms and upper back are strengthened.

It is my opinion that spinning has an effect on the water in the body. For many years I practiced and taught a form of bodywork called Holistic Pulsing, which was developed by Tovi Browning, an osteopath.

Holistic Pulsing uses a wide range of rocking motions directed at the water within the body—in the blood, muscles, bones, and brain. The rocking deliberately creates waves and oscillations, and uses the power of the water to dissolve blockages and release tension.

Since the body is more water than anything else—around 70 percent, in fact—I believe that spinning assists the flow of the waters of your body: your blood, cerebrospinal fluid, digestive juices, hormonal and lymphatic systems, etc. As you spin, you create vortexes (mini whirlpools) in the waters of your body (as in Holistic Pulsing), revitalizing it and helping to remove toxins.

Spinning also raises your energy. I call it Tibetan Caffeine! If you are tired and have to go out to dinner or get through the afternoon at work, try a spin. Follow it with three Energy Breaths (see page 34) and you will be calm, focused and raring to go.

Lastly, remember the truism "Like cures like." When your mind is spinning or full, it can be very therapeutic to do the Spin. It helps you stop "spinning out" and clears the fog out of your mind.

Above all—spinning is fun!

PREPARATION

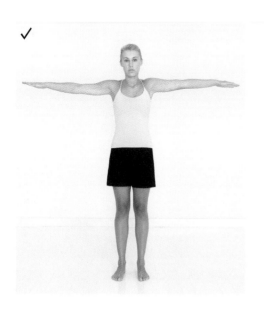

✓

1. **Caution**

   Begin turning slowly, as spinning can cause dizziness. It can also make some people feel a bit nauseous, lose balance or develop a headache. (It is important to build up your repetitions gradually.) If you have any of the conditions listed in Part 1 on pages 20–21, check with your doctor before attempting the Spin.

2. **Correct posture**

   Stand with your legs hip-width apart and unlock your knees. Make a strong connection to the earth underneath your feet and make certain your weight is evenly balanced between your feet. Keep your head level, looking straight ahead. Make sure your chin isn't sticking out. Imagine a string attached to the ceiling is pulling your whole body upright through the middle of your head.

   When you are ready, raise your arms up straight, like wings, beside you. If your shoulders are hunched, drop them down and back; your arms should be level with your normal shoulder height (see left).

3. **Foot positions**

   In the Beginners level of T5T, your right foot should remain in constant contact with the floor. This method helps you develop confidence in your spin by teaching you how to spin in one spot (without moving across the floor), and you can use your foot as a brake to help you slow down.

   Keep your right foot on the floor as you turn, sliding your right toes around as you step with your left foot.

   In the Intermediate/Advanced level, you release the foot, allowing both feet to move freely in a more dance-like motion.

4. **Stability and control**

   During the Spin, lightly engage your pelvic floor and lower abdominals. Keep your focus on a central point three finger-widths below your belly button, and initiate all your movement from this power center. This "inner reference" feels rather like holding on to a pole as you swing around it. This will stabilize your movement and help you to balance.

5. **Soft eyes and counting spins**

   Interestingly, when you focus intently, your breathing also narrows (restricts). Softening (unfocusing) your eyes expands your field of vision and your breathing. It also encourages a more relaxed spin. To count repetitions use a change of color; for example, a doorway. As you spin you will see this in your peripheral vision only. Count each time the color flashes past.

6. **Watch your speed**

As you build up repetitions, the momentum increases your speed. Start slowing down several repetitions before you intend to stop. If you don't, you may find yourself trying to stand upright while your body is still spinning.

Do not attempt to speed up your spin until you are certain of your ability to control the movement, and until you can remain in one spot. (Learning the Spin at the Beginners level will teach you how to do this—see page 62.)

If you have to change the focus of your eyes for any reason, you will find yourself unable to control your body and you will weave across the floor.

Be aware of children or animals in your presence. If you are spinning fast you may find it difficult to stop suddenly and you may trip over them!

7. **Remember to breathe**

During the First Rite, breathe in and out through the nose, taking normal and comfortable breaths. Most people forget to breathe in the early stages of learning the Spin, as they are concentrating on getting the movement correct.

Holding your breath or shallow breathing will cause tension in your body or reduce your oxygen supply. This is exactly what you want to avoid, as it will prevent you from experiencing a smooth, free and enjoyable spin.

8. **Stopping**

When you stop, close your eyes immediately. (Note: Some people find that leaving their eyes open helps reduce dizziness, while others prefer to close them.)

Stand with your legs hip-width apart and your knees slightly bent, and begin the Energy Breathing Technique (see page 34) immediately. Focus only on the breath, allowing your body to relax as you slowly breathe out.

To reduce dizziness, some people like to clasp their fingers together in front of them and focus on their thumbs until they feel okay again.

9. **Daily variations**

Your ability to spin is affected by your mental state on a day-to-day basis. If your mind is foggy, stressed or full, you will find it quite challenging to focus while practicing the Spin. However, once you start spinning and regain control of your thoughts, you will find that your mind has cleared and you will feel more centered and stable.

Be prepared for days when you will fly like a glider; others when you will clunk around, and so on. In the early stages of practicing the Spin, people often find that if they are "all over the place" during their spin, the rest of their day tends to shape up the same way! Later, with regular practice you will be able to carry the calm and focused benefits of the Five Rites through your day.

BEGINNERS

Remain at this level for week one. You will be doing three repetitions per day. When you have finished the Spin, turn to Solutions to Common Problems on pages 66–67 to see if there are changes you need to make. You need to fine-tune your movement until you are smooth, controlled and aerodynamic, before moving on to the Intermediate/Advanced level.

Your aims

To master the technique of the Spin and to achieve three repetitions; in particular:

- To achieve a smooth, graceful, even and balanced aerodynamic movement that feels easy and pleasurable.
- To be able to control the speed of your spin in both speeding up and in slowing down without losing smoothness.
- To be able to maintain your location without traveling across the floor.
- To be able to breathe naturally and rhythmically throughout the Spin, creating a delightfully free and flowing movement.

Instructions

1. Stand up straight with your legs hip-width apart. With your palms facing downward, raise your arms up straight, like wings, beside you.

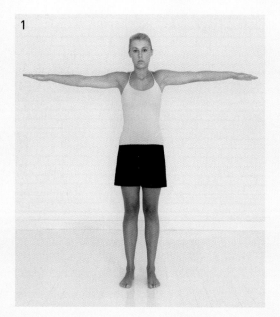

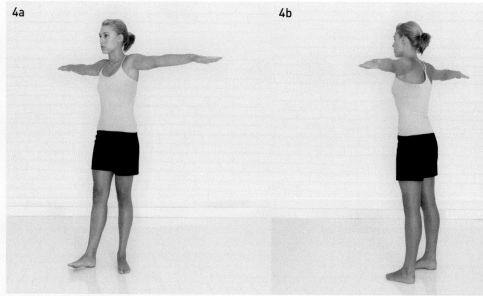

2. Pick an object with a change of color, for example, a doorway or a window ledge, to help you count your repetitions. (Every time you see this object you count a spin.)

3. Take a breath in through the nose to remind you to breathe. Continue to breathe comfortably and naturally through your nose, remembering to check on your breathing during the spin.

4. Keeping your right foot firmly on the floor, and with your arms outstretched and your head facing forward, start to turn from left to right in a clockwise direction, walking your left foot around your anchored right foot and spinning around in a complete circle.

5. Let your spin build up speed slowly and complete three spins in a steady, unbroken rhythm.

6. When you stop, immediately stand with your legs hip-width apart, knees slightly bent and your hands on your hips. Allow any dizziness to dissipate, then wrap your hands around your ribs in the Energy Breathing position. Breathe out then complete three Energy Breaths ending on an inhalation (see page 35, Step One). Wait until all dizziness disappears before beginning the Leg Raise.

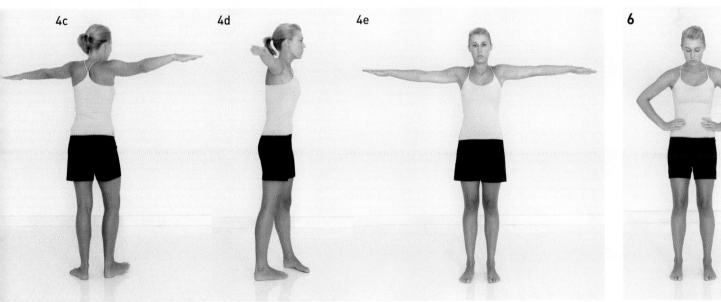

4c   4d   4e

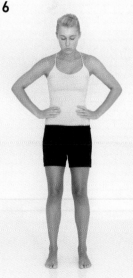

6

INTERMEDIATE/ADVANCED

The Intermediate and Advanced level of the Spin are the same. You begin this level at week two of your practice, when you have achieved all the outcomes of the Beginners level.

At this level you learn to spin with free feet and you build from three repetitions up to 21 repetitions per day.

Some people find that the foot movement described in the Intermediate/Advanced level helps them feel less dizzy. However, some people prefer to keep their right foot in constant contact with the floor. The benefits are the same, whichever method you choose.

Your aims

- To be able to move smoothly with both your feet stepping around in small circles as you spin.
- To build up to 21 repetitions.
- To maintain your position without wandering across the floor.

Note: If you are traveling across the floor, then you are not ready to move on to the Intermediate/Advanced level. Traveling across the floor can cause you to bump into, or knock over, things with your outspread arms. (If you look down quickly you can become very dizzy, and may even fall.)

Be aware that with your feet loose, you will spin faster. Remember to build your speed up slowly, and to allow some time to slow down your spin rate before you come to a stop.

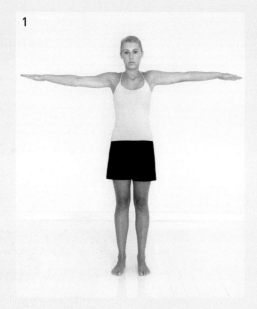

1

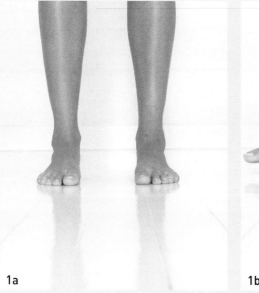

1a

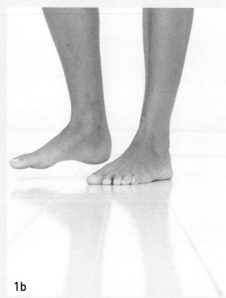

1b

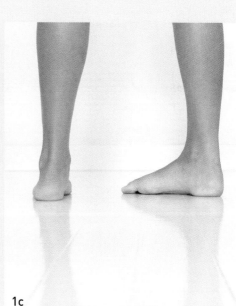

1c

Instructions

2

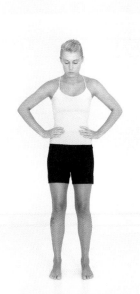

1. Follow the instructions for Beginners, but this time release your right foot and allow both feet to move freely around in a small circle as you spin. Concentrate on being loose and light on your feet, almost like a dancer.

2. After the required number of spins, come immediately into the bent-knee position. Move into the Energy Breathing position, then complete three Energy Breaths ending on an inhalation (see page 36, Step Two) and allow the dizziness to disappear before beginning the Leg Raise.

    If you are still suffering from dizziness after a number of weeks, see Solutions to Common Problems on page 66 or try some of the natural remedies and exercises on pages 68–69.

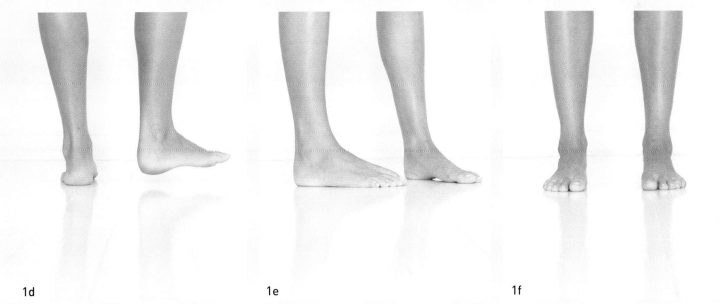

1d   1e   1f

SOLUTIONS TO COMMON PROBLEMS

1. Dizziness during the Rite or afterward

By far the greatest number of people experience very little to no dizziness when spinning if they follow the recommendation of the T5T program to build up repetitions slowly. If you do feel dizzy, the first step is to slow down. Next, check that your leg and arm movements are smooth and even, and then that your eye movements are steady. Lastly, are you breathing? If you are very stressed it may be difficult to relax. Use the visualization technique on page 68 to help you; holding a positive image in your mind rather than a negative image is essential.

If you are one of those people who do repeatedly feel a bit dizzy in the initial stages, even after just a few repetitions, be prepared to take it slowly. It is important not to go too fast too soon. Remember as you practice that any dizziness you have early on will most likely disappear with time. Refer to Natural Remedies for Dizziness on pages 68–69 for information on natural methods to help prevent dizziness.

The important thing is not to lose heart. The worst-case scenario is that you can still get great benefit by doing the Swinging Movement (see page 44) instead of the Spin, until your dizziness improves over time. Gradually start introducing one or two spins to see how you are progressing.

Most people find that the Energy Breathing Technique carried out between the Rites (see page 34) gives them the ability to rebalance themselves before commencing the Second Rite.

2. Tired arms

Doing the Spin naturally strengthens your arms, shoulders and neck. If you find it very difficult to hold your arms out straight for the required period of time, try slightly bending them to make it easier for you. Work toward eventually being able to hold your arms out straight. Be patient; your strength and tone will increase as you continue to practice.

3. Poor aerodynamics

a) Poor spin quality

A poor-quality spin travels across the floor instead of staying centered in one place. Check that your body and arm position are correct and that your foot movements are smooth and even. These should ensure that your spin does not wobble and that you have good speed entering and exiting.

b) Irregular foot movements

Check that your foot movements are smooth and comfortable, like a dance.

At the Beginners level, make sure the toes of your anchored right foot are barely off the floor. If you lift your toes too high (see left), you will end up

X

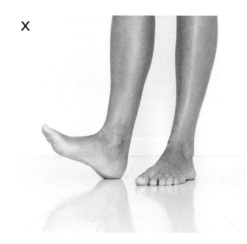

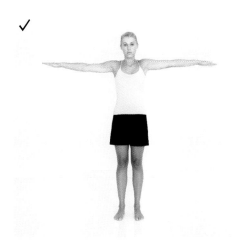
✓

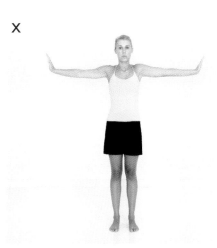
✗

pivoting on your heel. Your heel then becomes like the pointed tip of a spinning top, giving very little stability, control or smoothness to your movement. You are also at risk of toppling over!

Take comfortable and balanced steps. Tiny steps create a shaky, pneumatic-drill-like movement that can contribute to dizziness. Large, definite or uneven steps create a wobbly movement that can also make you feel dizzy.

If you have difficulty achieving smoothness, keep your arms by your sides and practice the foot movements on their own. (Note: Some people find that looking down at their feet makes them dizzy, so don't overdo it.)

c)   Uneven arms

If you have uneven arms, your movements will not be smooth and this may contribute to dizziness. Your arms are the force behind the turn and they help to keep your center tight. Make certain your arms are level (see top left). They should be held at the same height as your shoulders and your fingers should be together with palms facing downward, not pointing up (see middle left).

The most common mistake people make is having uneven arms (see below left). This causes imbalance and an unstable spin, which is particularly noticeable when you start to build up speed.

d)   Hunching your shoulders to your ears

People who hold a lot of tension in their neck and shoulders tend to hunch their shoulders toward their ears (see below). Others hunch them to compensate for a lack of strength in the arms. (Here they are recruiting the strong and overused upper back muscles to assist them in elevating their arms.) Relax and keep your shoulders back and down, but don't compress your spine. To keep your spine elongated, lift your breastbone but be careful not to arch your back; keep your arms level with your natural shoulder height.

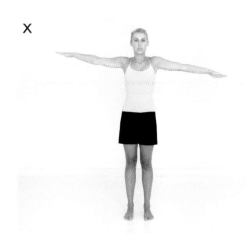
✗

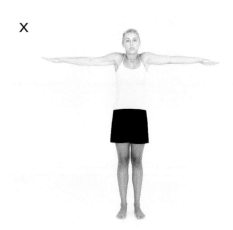
✗

FURTHER TIPS

Using visual metaphors

Using visualization can help you achieve your outcome. By holding an image in your mind of how you want to look, you will find it easier to achieve the movement you desire.

The Spin represents the element of energy. As you spin, you are creating a vortex of energy all the way up your spine, spinning each chakra as it moves upward toward your head and beyond. Imagine that you are controlling this vortex in a straight and uniform pattern—notice if you sway to the left, how the vortex of energy curves to the left with you like a child's Slinky toy. See yourself spinning more and more accurately so that you have a lovely vortex of energy swirling straight upward, gaining power and momentum with each perfect turn.

Another image that can help you achieve an aerodynamic spin is to imagine that you are an ice skater. Raise your arms on either side of your body, composing yourself, and then begin to spin. Imagine that you are cutting through the air with precision. You can feel the wind in your hair and upon your face as you start to spin faster. Now it's time for you to slow down. Imagine yourself coming to a graceful, even and smooth stop.

Curing dizziness
Why do we get dizzy?

There are many causes of dizziness. The dizziness referred to here is the motion sickness that some people experience in the early stages of practicing the Spin. If you experience dizziness you are not alone. Fortunately most people find that their symptoms improve with time and practice.

The symptoms of motion sickness occur because your brain receives conflicting information from your sensory systems. These senses send information to your brain about the position and movement of your body, and include your eyes, the sensors of the semicircular canals in your inner ears, and the somatosensory receptors in your skin, joints and muscles. A mismatch in sensory information causes a conflict between what is seen or felt and your previous orientational experience. When this happens, the body responds with the symptoms of dizziness and motion sickness. For this reason, using the correct technique during the Spin is crucial.

Natural remedies for dizziness

- Before you spin, drink a small glass of hot or cold water with some freshly squeezed lemon juice or a small slice of fresh ginger added. This often helps with nausea. Peppermint tea is also good for soothing the stomach.
- Take a supplement of Ginkgo biloba or feverfew. These may help prevent dizziness, but if you are taking medication check with your doctor first.
- Do not eat a heavy meal or drink alcoholic beverages before spinning.

- Spin in an area with plenty of fresh air—stuffy rooms do not help!
- After spinning, circle your fingers and thumb around your wrist approximately three finger-widths below the wrist folding line, between the flexor tendons. When you find a slightly tender spot, press your fingers into your arm (on the opposite side to your thumb). This point is called the Nei-Kuan pressure point. According to Traditional Chinese Medicine, pressure on this point has the effect of harmonizing and balancing the Yin and Yang of the *Qi* (life energy), so it can again flow unhindered. Pressing on this point can also help reduce motion sickness, dizziness and nausea—often within a few minutes.
- Limit your intake of salt and caffeine. They may impair the circulation of your blood, as will smoking.
- Learn to manage stress. Doing the Five Rites will greatly help with this.

Desensitizing exercises to help prevent dizziness

These exercises help strengthen your body's balance systems to enable you to spin. They can also be used to help prevent motion sickness.

- Slowly look up, and then look down. Repeat this movement several times while increasing the speed from slow to rapid. Now look from left to right, going from slow to fast as before. Repeat these eye movements several times a day.
- In a sitting or standing position, toss a tennis ball from hand to hand. Follow the arc of the ball with your eyes.
- Place a stable chair next to a wall so that you can reach out and touch it if needed. Sit on the chair with your feet flat on the floor. Focus your eyes on a target three to six meters (10 to 20 feet) away while you stand up slowly and then sit down again with your eyes open. Repeat this several times, then try the same exercise with your eyes closed (lightly touching the wall for security if and when needed).
- Clear a path next to a wall or behind a sofa. Walk backward and forward alongside the wall or sofa several times. Then, by holding on to the wall or the sofa, close your eyes and repeat the same exercise several times.

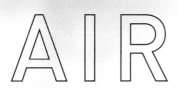

AIR

thinking, mental quickness,
clarity, intellect, breathing,
originality, versatility

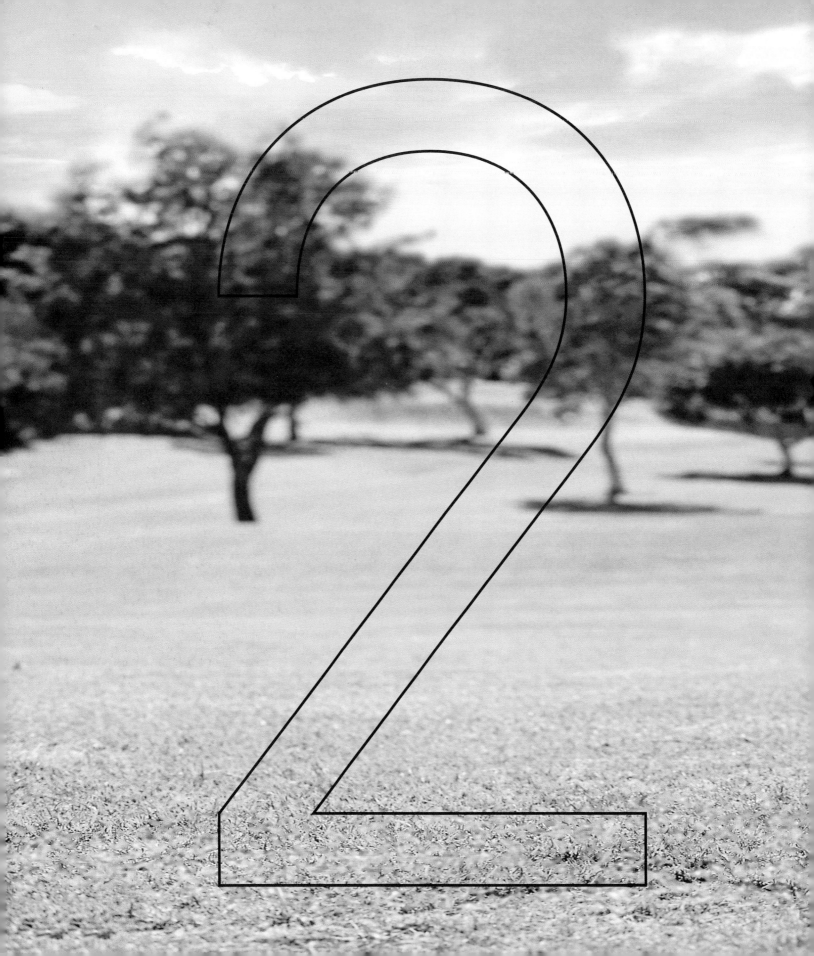

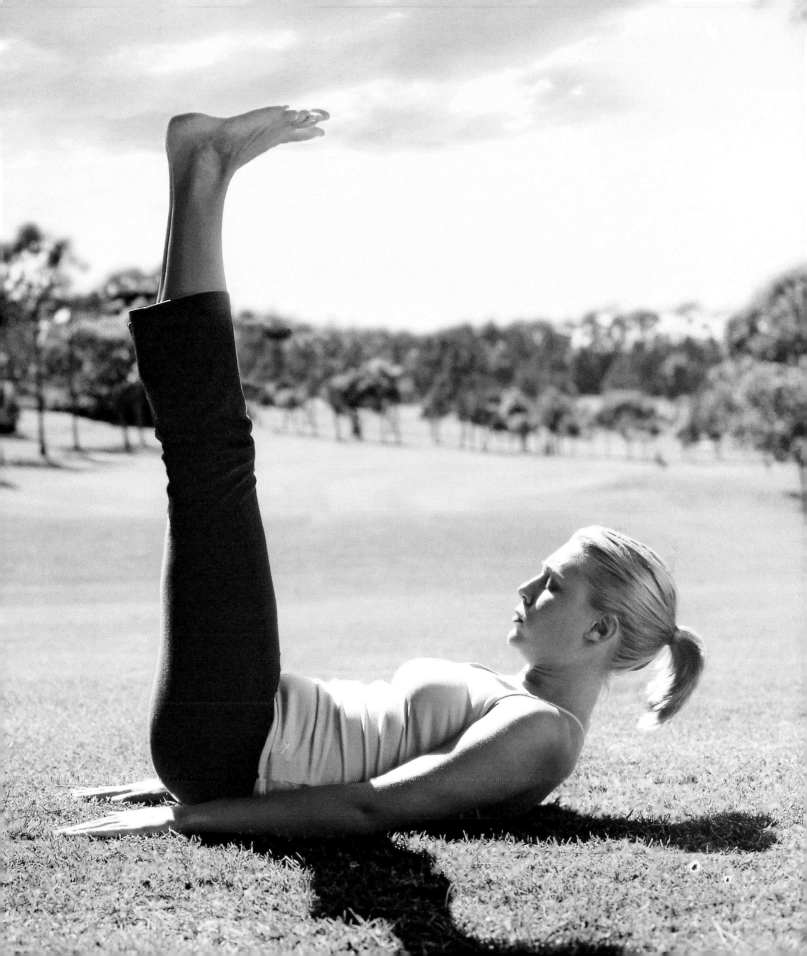

AIR The Leg Raise represents the need for clear, calm and focused thinking, utilizing the many health benefits of deep breathing and its ability to instill peace. As you do this practice, you learn to focus your mind in order to control the movement of specific muscle groups. A great synergy exists between the mind and the body. Imagine yourself as calm and focused, breathing deeply and able to perform each step with ease. Take this awareness into your normal life—that by breathing deeply and by maintaining a daily focus on your "bodymind," you can restore clarity and a razor-sharp focus in areas of confusion or stress in your life.

2ND RITE
THE LEG RAISE

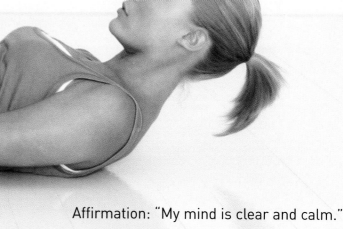

Affirmation: "My mind is clear and calm."

INTRODUCTION

It is good to have an end to journey toward; but it is the journey that matters in the end. Ursula K. Le Guin

Learning the Leg Raise involves by far the most steps (10) of the five Rites; the others have only two or three steps each. This gradual progression—by one step each week—enables your core stability muscles to develop the strength necessary to complete the final version of this posture. The last step will also bring you up to the full 21 repetitions you are aiming for.

The Leg Raise is not particularly difficult to perform, but you need to practice it with strength and control to minimize the risk of strain or injury. The forces involved in lifting your legs into position are strong, and your body must be correctly aligned and stabilized to assist your muscles in performing this movement optimally.

Benefits

In traditional yogic philosophy, inversions (the reverse of normal downward flow) are said to be the ultimate Fountain of Youth. Inversions are renowned for their age-reversing qualities, which is one of the reasons why advanced yoga practitioners practice headstands.

The effect of gravity is rather like an hourglass—whichever way you turn it, the contents always run toward the Earth. Over time, your body will have accumulated all sorts of waste products and impurities. When you invert your body, this reversal of gravity gives your circulatory system a helping hand.

In the Leg Raise you are combining an inversion with significant muscle strengthening. As your legs rise, you can feel the muscular contractions at various heights creating pressure: starting with your reproductive organs, up through your digestive organs, heart and lungs, your thyroid and into the brain. This contraction and relaxation of the muscles considerably improves blood flow around the body, including the flow to most of your internal organs and glands.

Raising your legs in T5T improves circulation and helps take the load off your veins. It stimulates your lymphatic system, which is dependent upon muscular movement and gravity, and is responsible for fluid balance (important for swollen legs), waste removal and the immune system.

The Leg Raise is a powerful and satisfying stretch for the hamstrings, calves, and Achilles. It strengthens and tones the muscles around your hips, abdomen, lower back, legs and neck and, in particular, powerfully strengthens your core stability muscles, helping you to develop a flatter stomach and protect your spine.

Holding the chin-to-chest position increases the work of the lower abdominal muscles, helping them to increase strength and provide stability for the spine. The cervical (neck) section of the spine is lengthened in a powerful stretch, helping to loosen tension and stiffness. This position also strengthens the neck and upper back.

The Leg Raise improves bowel and digestive functions. You may become more regular. Some people say it helps with menstrual cramps and irregular periods, although others find they need to reduce repetitions during menstruation.

PREPARATION

1. **Caution**

If you have any of the conditions listed in Part 1 on pages 20–21 or if you have retinal or eye-pressure (glaucoma) problems or a hiatal hernia, or have had recent abdominal surgery, you need to gain your doctor's approval before attempting the Leg Raise. Take this book with you to make assessment easier.

If you have excessive tension in the shoulders or legs or have weak abdominal muscles, do the Leg Raise very slowly and increase your repetitions by only one or two per week.

If you are menstruating, this Rite may interrupt your period or aggravate (or improve) cramping.

2. **Before you begin**

Before you attempt the Leg Raise, make certain that you have read and completed the exercises in Part 2 (see pages 25–44). In particular you will need to understand and be able to perform the lifting "up and in" of your core stability muscles combined with breathing wide into your ribs and back.

3. **Finding your neutral spine**

You will also need to be able to find your neutral spine. Neutral spine is when your back is supported in a neutral (normal) position, where the natural curves of your back are maintained; your hips should not be tilted up or down and your sacrum should rest squarely on the floor.

To find your neutral spine, follow the instructions below.

Exercise

X

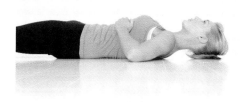

- Lie on your back with your legs straight. Place a small towel underneath your head to align it with your spine. Your lower back should be neither arched nor flattened against the floor. There should be just a small gap between the floor and your lower back.

X

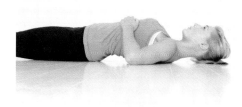

- Imagine north is your head and south your feet. Gently tilt your pelvis to the north, noticing how you lose the curve in your lower back as your waist gets pressed back to the floor (see top left).

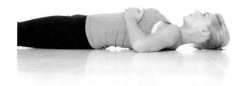

- Now gently tip your pelvis to the south, noticing how your lower back overarches (see middle left). (Do this step carefully and if you feel any discomfort, stop. Seek the advice of a medical professional before continuing.)
- Find the midpoint between these two extremes. Also make certain that your pelvis is level east to west. Tilt your hips to the right and to the left to find this midpoint. (See bottom left).

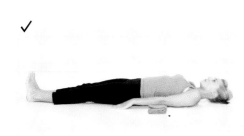

Throughout the Leg Raise, keep your spine in neutral, paying particular attention to avoid tilting the pelvis north. Maintaining a neutral spine throughout the movement will work your deep abdominals to provide good core stability.

4. **Equipment**

You will need a small bath towel for the Leg Raise (see left).

Before you perform the Leg Raise, place the towel, folded to about the thickness of your hand, in the hollow of your lower back. Spend some time working out the most comfortable thickness of towel for you to maintain a neutral spine.

5. **Imprinting the spine**

When raising or lowering your torso off or onto the floor, try to make contact with the floor vertebra by vertebra as you curl your spine. Imagine your spine is like a string of pearls being lowered or raised one by one. This will keep your spine supple and strong and prevent any jerky movements.

6. **Strength development**

Do only the number of repetitions that can be done without fatiguing your lower abdominals or back. It is important to listen to your body and to do only the number of repetitions that is comfortable. The Leg Raise is a particularly dynamic Rite, especially at the Advanced level, and must be taken at your own pace.

Warm-up
Knees-to-chest squeeze

This movement stretches and releases tension in your lower back, sacrum and hips in preparation for the Leg Raise.

Exercise

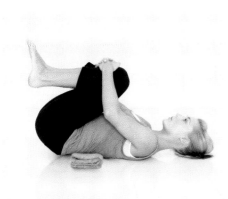

- Lie on the floor on your back with your knees bent and hip-width apart.
- Bring one knee toward your chest, then the other. Place your hands around your knees (or shins) and gently pull them toward your chest (see left).
- Breathe out and relax your spine, shoulders, neck and head onto the floor. Relax your hips and allow your knees to drop further toward your chest. To further release your back, make small circular movements with your knees (or rock side to side), gently massaging your sacrum and the back muscles on either side of your spine. Do this for about 10 seconds.

You are now ready to begin the Leg Raise. If you find you need a little fine tuning along the way, turn to pages 94–95, for Solutions to Common Problems.

BEGINNERS

STEP ONE

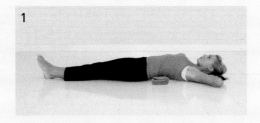

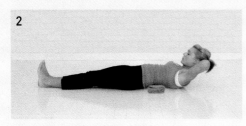

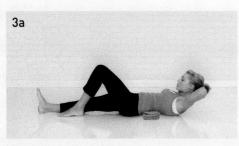

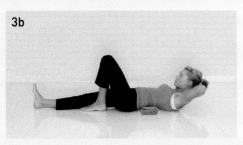

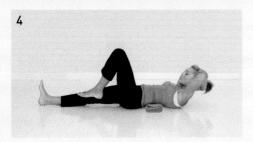

The Leg Raise is learned by following a series of steps at each of the Beginners, Intermediate and Advanced levels. These steps encourage a progressive buildup of strength in your core stability muscles to enable you to safely complete the final version of the posture. They also ensure correct technique, which is essential to minimize strain on the neck, back and abdomen. An extra step is added each week until the tenth week, when you will be doing 21 repetitions of the Advanced posture.

SINGLE BENT-LEG RAISE WITH HANDS BEHIND HEAD

This is essentially your introduction to the Leg Raise. Perform the Rite at this basic level for the first week, or until you are able to do three repetitions.

Your aims

To learn the mechanical requirements of the Leg Raise—starting position, chin-to-chest position, leg raise, full leg extension, leg return—using a single bent leg.

Instructions

Note: You don't need a pillow under your head for this step, as you will be using your arms to support your head.

1. Lie on your back in the neutral spine position with a towel under your lower back (see Preparation, page 77). Make sure your shoulders are relaxed and not hunched, and that you are lying straight.

    Lace your fingers together and place them under the base of your skull. Let your elbows sit forward to allow your upper back muscles to remain relaxed and to help you maintain your abdominal focus throughout the movement.

    "Soften" your throat, making sure it is not compressed by the chin being too far forward, or stretched by the chin being too far backward.

    Lift your pelvic floor and pull your lower abdominals in toward your spine—maintain this throughout the entire movement. Keep your focus on your lower abdomen and move from this central core throughout the movement.

2. Breathe in, expanding the ribs wide to the sides and into the back, and at the same time use your stomach muscles (*not* your arms) to lift your head. Rotate your chin toward your neck, then chest—the lower part of your shoulder blades and rib cage should remain in contact with the floor. Look at your belly button and do not allow your lower abdominals to bulge outward (they must stay flattened toward your spine). Once in this position hold your breath.

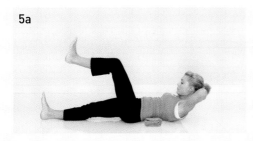

5a

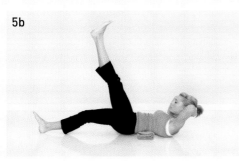

5b

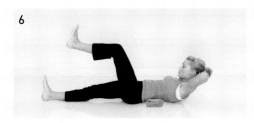

6

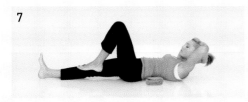

7

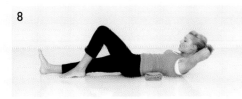

8

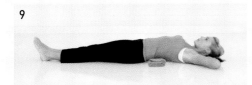

9

3. Bend your right knee and slide your foot along the floor to your bottom.

4. Lift your knee until it is directly over your hip: you are aiming for a 90-degree angle between your thigh and body. Make sure your kneecap is not rotated outward or inward: it should be centered.

5. Carefully maintaining this thigh position (knee over hip), raise your foot and straighten your leg toward the ceiling, but don't lock your knee. You are aiming to straighten your raised leg until it is perpendicular to your body, but this may take some time to achieve. (In the initial stages it is more important to maintain core stability and keep your sacrum pressed to the floor. Work toward being able to straighten and fully raise your leg over time.) Flex your toes and visualize your entire leg lengthening.

6. Breathe out, keeping your pelvic floor lifted and your lower abdominals pulled in toward your spine, while you bend your knee back down into the 90-degree position. (As you begin to lower your foot, begin to lower your head—returning it to the floor in a smooth and controlled manner, feeling each vertebra pressing one at a time into the floor beneath you. Continue this throughout the following moments, until your head touches the floor just after your leg comes to rest.)

7. Lower your thigh, bringing your heel back toward your buttock.

8. Let your foot touch the floor and then slide your leg along the floor until it is straight. Your breath out should correspond to your leg coming down, being completed by the time your leg is again resting on the floor.

9. Allow all your muscles to relax, then repeat the above steps using your left leg. When you have completed this cycle you have performed one repetition.

10. Repeat this exercise in a steady, unbroken rhythm for three repetitions.

11. Remain lying on your back, bend your knees and place your hands in the Energy Breathing Position with your hands wrapped around your lower ribs.
    Exhale fully, then take three complete Energy Breaths ending on an inhalation (see page 35, Step One).

To get into the starting position for the Kneeling Backbend, roll your hips and shoulders *together* onto your right side and push yourself up using your right elbow and your left hand. Come onto your knees in the prayer position.

STEP **TWO**

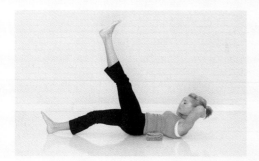

SINGLE BENT-LEG RAISE WITH HANDS BEHIND HEAD—SYNCHRONIZING BREATHING WITH MOVEMENT

During the previous movement you learned to take a breath while you moved your chin toward your chest and then to hold your breath as you raised your leg. In Step Two, you maintain a long inhalation while simultaneously lifting your head and leg. In this way, the movement and the breath become synchronized.

Perform this step for one week (week two of your program) or until you are able to do five repetitions.

Your aims

To synchronize the raising of the head and leg with breathing. And to maintain smoothness and control of the movement.

Instructions

Note: You don't need a pillow under your head for this step, as you will be using your arms to support your head.

If you run out of breath before your leg is in the upright position don't try to compensate by rushing the movement to keep pace with the breath, which can make you lose control and jerk your neck or flick your leg into position.

The solution is to breathe in deeply and slowly, expanding the ribs wide to the sides and into the back. Breathe out as you bring your leg back down again. Complete exhaling by the time your leg is brought back to the floor and let your head be the last part of your body to touch the floor.

1.   Lie on your back in the neutral spine position with a towel under your lower back.

Lace your fingers together, and place them under the base of your skull. "Soften" your throat.

Lift your pelvic floor and pull your lower abdominals in toward your spine. Keep your focus on your lower abdomen and move from this central core throughout the movement.

2.   Breathe in through your nose as you lift your chin toward your chest. At the same time, slide your right foot along the ground toward your buttocks, raise your thigh to 90 degrees and straighten your leg until perpendicular to your body.

Flex your toes. If your legs remain bent, work toward gradually being able to straighten them over time.

3. Check that your lower abdominals and pelvic floor are engaged, and breathe out through your nose as you bend your knee to the 90-degree position, return your foot to the floor, then slide your foot along the floor until your leg is straight. (You should have completed exhaling by the time your leg is on the floor.) As you lower your foot, lower your head—returning it to the floor in a smooth and controlled manner, feeling each vertebra pressing one at a time into the floor beneath you.

4. Allow all your muscles to relax, then repeat the above steps, raising and lowering the left leg. When you have completed this cycle you have performed one repetition.

5. Repeat this exercise in a steady, unbroken rhythm for five repetitions.

6. Remain lying on your back, bend your knees and place your hands in the Energy Breathing Position with your hands wrapped around your lower ribs.

Exhale fully, then take three complete Energy Breaths ending on an inhalation (see page 36, Step Two).

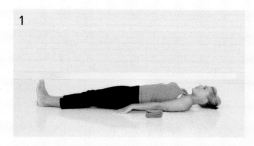

1

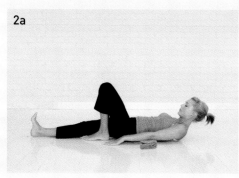

2a

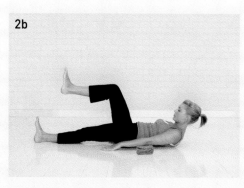

2b

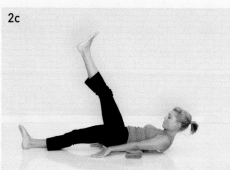

2c

SINGLE BENT-LEG RAISE
WITH ARMS BY SIDES

This step is the same as Step Two but is performed with your hands by your sides.

Perform this step for one week (week three of your program) or until you are doing seven repetitions.

Test your neck strength and comfort first

Because your neck is unsupported in this movement, it is important to first test whether your neck is strong enough for you to perform the Rite without any discomfort developing.

The best way to do this is to practice Step Three first without the leg movement. This helps you discover how to lift your neck correctly and identifies any area of strain.

For this exercise, focus on using your abdominal muscles to lift your head. Do not use your arms. Do not use the momentum of the movement by flicking or jerking upright.

Exercise

- **Lie on your back with your arms by your sides, palms downward.**
- **Lift your pelvic floor and pull your lower abdominals in toward your spine.**
- **Breathe in as you slowly lift your chin toward your chest. Hold for five counts.**
- **Breathe out as you gently roll each vertebra back onto the floor.**

If you are able to do each of the steps above without any discomfort, you are ready to begin. If not, repeat these steps until you are confident that you are using the right muscles.

Your aims

To be able to bring your head off the floor in a straight, smooth and controlled movement, without pushing yourself up with your hands or jerking or skewing from one side to the other.

Instructions

Note: If your chin tilts backward when you are lying down, place a small towel underneath your head to keep your neck correctly aligned (see page 94). If you feel any strain in the neck, consider propping up your head with a firm pillow or books (see page 94).

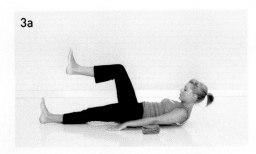

3a

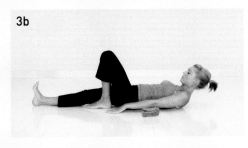

3b

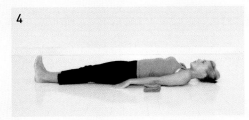

4

1. Lie on your back in the neutral spine position with a towel under your lower back and your arms by your sides, fingers together. Make sure you are lying straight and your head is not tilted to one side. "Soften" your throat by aligning your head with your spine.

   Lift your pelvic floor and pull your lower abdominals in toward your spine. Keep your focus on your lower abdomen and move from this central core throughout the movement.

2. Breathe in as you use your stomach muscles to slowly lift the top part of your shoulders off the floor and to bring your chin toward your chest (do not jerk or rock the shoulders and chin upward). At the same time, slide your right leg along the ground to your buttocks, raise your thigh to 90 degrees, then straighten your leg.

   Flex your toes. If your leg remains bent, work toward gradually being able to straighten it over time.

3. Check that your lower abdominals and pelvic floor are engaged, and breathe out through your nose as you bend your right knee to the 90-degree position, return your foot to the floor, then slide your foot along the floor until your leg is straight. (You should have completed exhaling by the time your leg is on the floor.) As you lower your foot, lower your head—returning it to the floor in a smooth and controlled manner, feeling each vertebra pressing one at a time into the floor beneath you.

4. Allow all your muscles to relax, then repeat the above steps, raising and lowering the left leg. When you have completed this cycle you have performed one repetition.

5. Repeat this exercise in a steady, unbroken rhythm for seven repetitions.

6. Remain lying on your back, bend your knees and place your hands in the Energy Breathing Position with your hands wrapped around your lower ribs.

   Exhale fully, then take three complete Energy Breaths ending on an inhalation (see page 36, Step Three).

STEP FOUR

The Intermediate level introduces the concept of performing the Leg Raise with both legs at the same time.

DOUBLE BENT-LEG RAISE

This step is the same as Step Three, but is performed with both legs at the same time.

Perform this step for one week (week four of your program) or until you are doing nine repetitions.

Your aims

To make certain your pelvis is completely immobilized. And to be able to perform the movement without rocking as you lift your legs up and down.

Instructions

1. Lie on your back in the neutral spine position with a towel under your lower back and your arms by your sides. Make sure you are lying straight and your head is not tilted to one side. "Soften" your throat by aligning your head with your spine.

    Lift your pelvic floor and pull your lower abdominals in toward your spine. Keep your focus on your lower abdomen and move from this central core throughout the movement.

2. Breathe in through your nose as you lift your chin toward your chest. At the same time, slide both feet along the ground toward your buttocks, press your thighs together as you raise them to 90 degrees and straighten your legs until

1

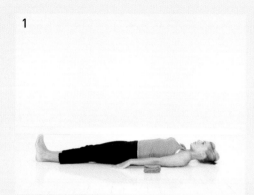

2a

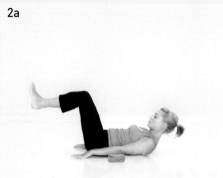

2b

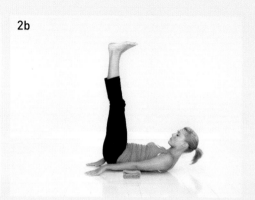

perpendicular to your body. Flex your toes. Make sure that you do not jerk your legs back across your body, lifting your tailbone off the floor. Make sure, also, that your pelvis is immobilized when bringing the legs up *and* down.

If your legs remain bent, work toward gradually being able to straighten them over time.

3. Check that your lower abdominals and pelvic floor are engaged, and breathe out as you bend your knees to the 90-degree position, return your feet to the floor and slide your feet along the floor until your legs are straight. As you lower your feet, lower your head—returning it to the floor in a smooth and controlled manner, feeling each vertebra pressing one at a time into the floor.

4. Allow all your muscles to relax. When you have completed this cycle you have performed one repetition.

5. Repeat this exercise in a steady, unbroken rhythm for nine repetitions.

6. Remain lying on your back, bend your knees and place your hands in the Energy Breathing Position with your hands wrapped around your lower ribs.

Exhale fully, then take three complete Energy Breaths ending on an inhalation (see page 36, Step Three).

3

4

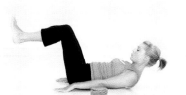

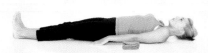

ADVANCED

STEP FIVE

At the Advanced level, straight-leg upward and downward movements are introduced a little at a time, until you are performing the ultimate double straight-leg Leg Raise.

SINGLE BENT-LEG RAISE WITH PARTIAL STRAIGHT-LEG DOWNWARD MOVEMENT

Perform this step for one week (week five of your program) or until you are doing 11 repetitions.

Your aims

To be able to fully control the pelvic floor, immobilizing your pelvis as you keep your leg straight and lower it *one third of the way* to the floor.

Instructions

1. Lie on your back in the neutral spine position with a towel under your lower back and your arms by your sides. Make sure you are lying straight and your head is not tilted to one side. "Soften" your throat by aligning your head with your spine.

    Lift your pelvic floor and pull your lower abdominals in toward your spine. Keep your focus on your lower abdomen and move from this central core throughout the movement.

1   2a   2b

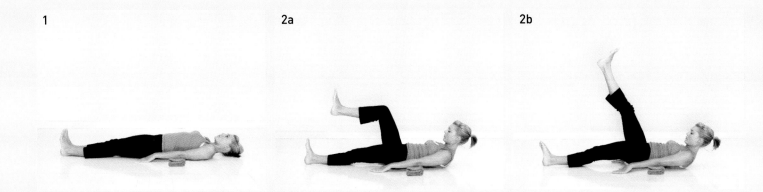

2. Breathe in through your nose as you lift your chin toward your chest. At the same time, slide your right foot along the ground toward your buttocks, raise your thigh to 90 degrees and straighten your leg until perpendicular to your body.

   Flex your toes. If your leg remains bent, work toward gradually being able to straighten it over time.

3. Check that your lower abdominals and pelvic floor are engaged, and breathe out—but instead of bending the knee again and bringing the foot toward the buttock, slowly bring the leg down straight one-third of the way to the floor.

4. At the one-third mark, bend your knee so that your foot touches the floor. Then slide your foot along the floor until the leg is straight. As you lower your leg, lower your head—returning it to the floor in a smooth and controlled manner, feeling each vertebra pressing one at a time into the floor beneath you.

5. Allow all your muscles to relax, then repeat the above step, raising and lowering the left leg. When you have completed this cycle you have performed one repetition.

6. Repeat this exercise in a steady, unbroken rhythm for 11 repetitions.

7. Remain lying on your back, bend your knees and place your hands in the Energy Breathing Position with your hands wrapped around your lower ribs.

   Exhale fully, then take three complete Energy Breaths ending on an inhalation (see page 36, Step Three).

3   4   5

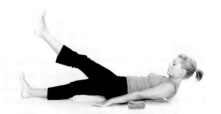
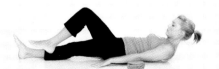
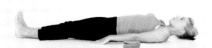

1

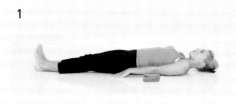

2a

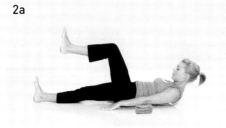

2b

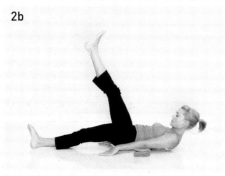

3

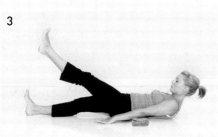

4

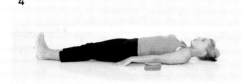

SINGLE BENT-LEG RAISE WITH FULL STRAIGHT-LEG DOWNWARD MOVEMENT

Perform this step for one week (week six of your program) or until you are doing 13 repetitions.

Your aims

To be able to fully control the pelvic floor, immobilizing your pelvis as you bring your straight leg *all the way* down to the floor.

Instructions

1. Lie on your back in the neutral spine position with a towel under your lower back and your arms by your sides. Make sure you are lying straight and your head is not tilted to one side. "Soften" your throat by aligning your head with your spine.

    Lift your pelvic floor and pull your lower abdominals in toward your spine. Keep your focus on your lower abdomen and move from this central core throughout the movement.

2. Breathe in through your nose as you lift your chin toward your chest. At the same time, slide your right foot along the ground toward your buttocks, raise your thigh to 90 degrees and straighten your leg until perpendicular to your body. Straighten your leg as much as possible and flex your toes.

3. Check that your lower abdominals and pelvic floor are engaged, and breathe out as you bring your leg *down straight all the way to the floor*. As you lower your leg, lower your head—returning it to the floor in a smooth and controlled manner, feeling each vertebra pressing one at a time into the floor beneath you.

4. Allow all your muscles to relax, then repeat the above steps, using the left leg. When you have completed this cycle you have performed one repetition.

5. Repeat this exercise in a steady, unbroken rhythm for 13 repetitions.

6. Remain lying on your back, bend your knees and place your hands in the Energy Breathing Position with your hands wrapped around your lower ribs.

    Exhale fully, then take three complete Energy Breaths ending on an inhalation (see page 36, Step Three).

SINGLE STRAIGHT-LEG RAISE

Perform this step for one week (week seven of your program) or until you are completing 15 repetitions.

Your aims

To be able to fully control the pelvic floor, immobilizing your pelvis as you raise and lower your straight leg.

Instructions

1. Lie on your back in the neutral spine position with a towel under your lower back and your arms by your sides. Make sure you are lying straight and your head is not tilted to one side. "Soften" your throat by aligning your head with your spine.

    Lift your pelvic floor and pull your lower abdominals in toward your spine. Keep your focus on your lower abdomen and move from this central core throughout the movement.

2. Breathe in through your nose as you lift your chin toward your chest. At the same time, *lift your straight right leg upward* until perpendicular to your body. Make certain your pelvis is immobilized and your tailbone does not lift off the floor.

    Keep your toes flexed throughout the movement. If your leg remains bent, work toward gradually being able to straighten it over time.

3. Check that your lower abdominals and pelvic floor are engaged, and breathe out as you bring your leg *down straight all the way to the floor.* As you lower your leg, lower your head—returning it to the floor in a smooth and controlled manner, feeling each vertebra pressing one at a time into the floor beneath you.

4. Allow all your muscles to relax, then repeat the above step, raising the left leg. When you have completed this cycle you have performed one repetition.

5. Repeat this exercise in a steady, unbroken rhythm for 15 repetitions.

6. Remain lying on your back, bend your knees and place your hands in the Energy Breathing Position with your hands wrapped around your lower ribs.

    Exhale fully, then take three complete Energy Breaths ending on an inhalation (see page 36, Step Three).

1

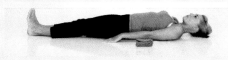

2a

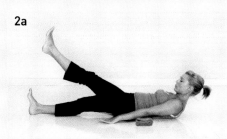

2b

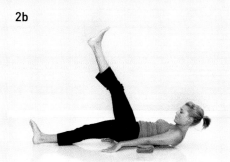

3

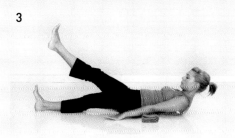

4

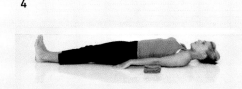

STEP EIGHT

DOUBLE BENT-LEG RAISE WITH PARTIAL STRAIGHT-LEG DOWNWARD MOVEMENT

Step Eight sees the introduction of double legs in combination with straight-leg downward movement.

Perform this step for one week (week eight of your program) or until you are doing 17 repetitions.

Your aims

To make certain that your legs come down to the midway point in a straight line—during this downward movement some people have a tendency to skew from one side to the other.

Instructions

1. Lie on your back in the neutral spine position with a towel under your lower back and your arms by your sides. Make sure you are lying straight and your head is not tilted to one side. "Soften" your throat by aligning your head with your spine.

    Lift your pelvic floor and pull your lower abdominals in toward your spine. Keep your focus on your lower abdomen and move from this central core throughout the movement.

2. Breathe in through your nose as you lift your chin toward your chest. At the same time, slide both feet along the ground toward your buttocks, raise your thighs to 90 degrees and straighten your legs until perpendicular to your body.

1

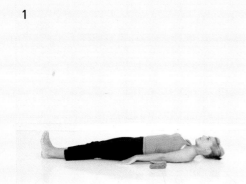

2a

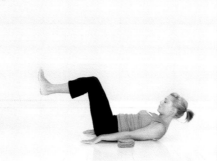

2b

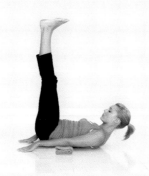

Make sure that you do not jerk your legs back across your body, lifting your tailbone off the floor. Make sure, also, that your pelvis is immobilized when bringing the legs up *and* down.

Straighten your legs as much as possible, keeping your toes flexed and legs pressed together throughout the movement. The aim is to get your legs as straight as possible without lifting your tailbone off the floor. If you have to bend your knees, work toward eventually being able to straighten your legs over time.

3.   Check that your lower abdominals and pelvic floor are engaged, and breathe out as you slowly bring your legs *down straight one-third of the way to the floor.*

4.   At the one-third mark, bend your knees so that your feet touch the floor. Then slide your feet along the floor until your legs are straight. As you lower your legs, lower your head—returning it to the floor in a smooth and controlled manner, feeling each vertebra pressing one at a time into the floor beneath you.

5.   Allow all your muscles to relax. When you have completed this cycle you have performed one repetition.

6.   Repeat this exercise in a steady, unbroken rhythm for 17 repetitions.

7.   Remain lying on your back, bend your knees and place your hands in the Energy Breathing Position with your hands wrapped around your lower ribs.

Exhale fully, then take three complete Energy Breaths ending on an inhalation (see page 36, Step Three).

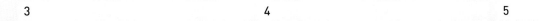

3   4   5

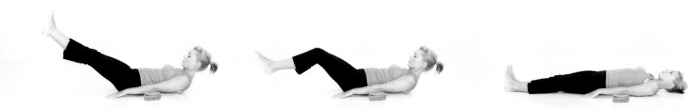

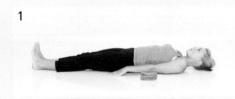

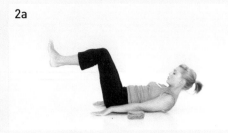

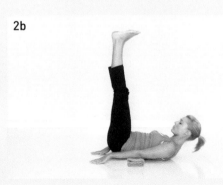

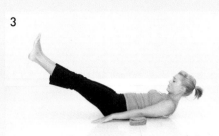

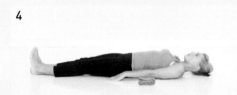

DOUBLE BENT-LEG RAISE WITH FULL STRAIGHT-LEG DOWNWARD MOVEMENT

In this step, both legs are brought down straight all the way to the floor.

Perform this step for one week (week nine of your program) or until you are doing 19 repetitions.

Your aims

To make certain that your legs come down to the floor in a straight line, and your pelvis remains immobilized with your sacrum pressed to the floor.

Instructions

1. Lie on your back in the neutral spine position with a towel under your lower back and your arms by your sides. Make sure you are lying straight. "Soften" your throat by aligning your head with your spine. Lift your pelvic floor and pull your lower abdominals in toward your spine. Keep your focus on your lower abdomen and move from this central core throughout the movement.

2. Breathe in through your nose as you lift your chin toward your chest. At the same time, slide both feet along the ground toward your buttocks, raise your thighs to 90 degrees and straighten your legs until perpendicular to your body. Make sure your pelvis is immobilized when bringing the legs up *and* down.

   Keep your toes flexed and your legs pressed together throughout the movement.

3. Check that your lower abdominals and pelvic floor are engaged, and breathe out as you bring *both legs down straight all the way to the floor*. As you lower your legs, lower your head—returning it to the floor in a smooth and controlled manner, feeling each vertebra pressing one at a time into the floor beneath you.

4. Allow all your muscles to relax. When you have completed this cycle you have performed one repetition.

5. Repeat this exercise in a steady, unbroken rhythm for 19 repetitions.

6. Remain lying on your back, bend your knees and place your hands in the Energy Breathing Position with your hands wrapped around your lower ribs.

   Exhale fully, then take three complete Energy Breaths ending on an inhalation (see page 36, Step Three).

DOUBLE STRAIGHT-LEG RAISE

In this step, both legs are straight and are pressed tightly together as you raise them up and down.

Congratulations, you've made it to 21 repetitions and the full version of this detailed Rite!

1

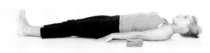

Your aims

To make certain as your legs come up and down that they stay together and travel in a straight line from the top of the movement to the bottom of the movement and vice versa (and don't skew from side to side).

2a

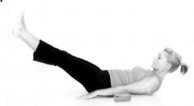

Instructions

1.   Lie on your back in the neutral spine position with a towel under your lower back and your arms by your sides. Press your legs together so they operate as one.

Lift your pelvic floor and pull your lower abdominals in toward your spine.

2b

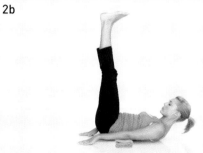

2.   Breathe in through your nose as you lift your chin toward your chest. At the same time, lift both legs straight upward, keeping them pressed together, until perpendicular to your body. Make certain that your pelvis is immobilized and your tailbone does not lift off the floor.

Keep your toes flexed and your legs pressed together throughout the movement.

3.   Check that your lower abdominals and pelvic floor are engaged, and breathe out as you bring both legs, pressed together, straight down all the way to the floor. As you lower your legs, lower your head—returning it to the floor in a smooth and controlled manner, feeling each vertebra pressing one at a time into the floor beneath you.

3

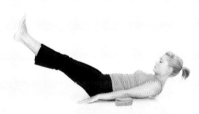

4.   Allow all your muscles to relax, and repeat this exercise in a steady, unbroken rhythm for 21 repetitions.

5.   Remain lying on your back, bend your knees and place your hands in the Energy Breathing Position with your hands wrapped around your lower ribs.

Exhale fully, then take three complete Energy Breaths ending on an inhalation (see page 36, Step Three).

4

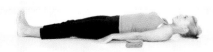

SOLUTIONS TO COMMON PROBLEMS

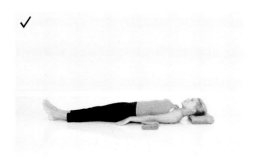

✓

1. **Lying crooked**

   Lying with your body at an angle affects the symmetry of your movement. This creates muscle imbalance and places uneven pressure on your joints, ligaments and tendons. Check that you are lying straight before you begin.

2. **Moving crooked**

   Due to unequal strength between the left and the right sides of our body, some people incorrectly skew to the left or the right as they raise their torso off the ground. Others are fine with the torso movement, but when they lift their chin toward their chest they tilt their head to one side. As mentioned above, this skewing to one side places uneven pressure on your muscles, joints, ligaments and tendons.

   If you experience this, before you begin the Leg Raise, line yourself up with a vertical line, such as the edge of a window or picture frame. As you raise your head, torso and legs, make certain that your movement is straight.

3. **Incorrect head position**

   If your chin tilts backward when you lie flat on the floor, place a small folded towel under your head (see left). Your head and neck should be aligned with your spine and your throat should be soft, not stretched or compressed.

4. **Weak neck**

   Always rest your head when your neck becomes tired. If you have a weak neck, try forestalling muscle fatigue by resting your head on something firm, such as a few books. The higher your head is raised, the shorter the distance to lift your chin to your chest. You can either leave your head resting on the books as you do the exercise, or you can continue to perform the chin-to-chest position. As your neck strength increases, remove one book at a time, until your head is resting on the floor (or a towel).

5. **Jerking and flicking**

   Due to muscle imbalances and weakness, some people use the momentum of the movement to lift their head and feet up and down. This puts them at risk of strain or injury. Make certain your movement is smooth and controlled by raising and lowering your spine vertebra by vertebra as explained in Imprinting the Spine (see page 77).

   Erratic movements can also be the result of fatigue, not using your core stability muscles, or holding your breath when you should be breathing. If any of these problems are the case, stop or do fewer repetitions. Give your body time to develop strength.

6. Rocking pelvis

Your pelvis *must* remain immobilized throughout the movement. It must not rock from side to side, but should remain stationary at all times.

7. Lifting your tailbone off the floor

When raised, your legs should not extend back over the abdomen at all, as this lifts your tailbone off the ground. Raise them just to the point where they are in line with your hips. Your sacrum should be pressed down to the floor at all times in the Leg Raise, to maintain a neutral spine and to provide core stability.

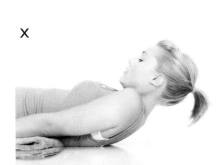

8. Using your hands to push yourself off the floor

Your arms are useful to stabilize and balance you, but you should not use them to push yourself off the floor. This is often done to compensate for weak core abdominal muscles, while the aim of T5T is to strengthen your core muscles so that your spine is protected. You won't get strong core stability muscles using your arms in this way—just strong arms!

9. Hunched shoulders

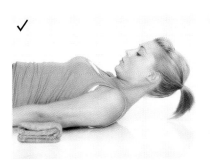

It is a common mistake to tense the shoulders, pulling them up toward your ears as you perform this movement (see top left). To avoid this, in the starting position press your shoulder blades down and backward onto the floor. Bring your chin toward your chest by rotating it forward from your jaw (see middle left).

10. Bent legs

Due to muscle tightness in the hamstrings and calf muscles, you may not be able to straighten your legs (see left). In the Leg Raise it is more important to keep the pelvis immobilized and to maintain neutral spine than it is to straighten the legs.

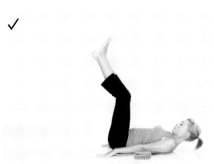

Raise your legs only until you feel a comfortable stretch, even if you are flexible. Work toward being able to straighten them eventually, but be patient with yourself and give yourself time.

FURTHER TIPS

Visual metaphors

Visual metaphors can often help people perform the Rites correctly. One of the following images might help you with the Leg Raise.

The crane

Imagine that you are a crane lifting a heavy weight. Your legs are the boom carrying the heavy weight and your torso is the crane's foundation. Imagine your crane firmly anchored to the ground, its foundations evenly balanced, smoothly swinging the boom (your legs) with complete control.

The torch beam

Imagine that on each of your hipbones there is a torch shining a beam up to the ceiling. Focus on keeping the beam strong and steady during the whole movement, instead of letting it wave around.

The marvelous richness of human experience would lose something of rewarding joy if there were no limitations to overcome. The hilltop hour would not be half so wonderful if there were no dark valleys to traverse. Helen Keller, 1880–1968, blind and deaf author, lecturer and model of disabled achievement

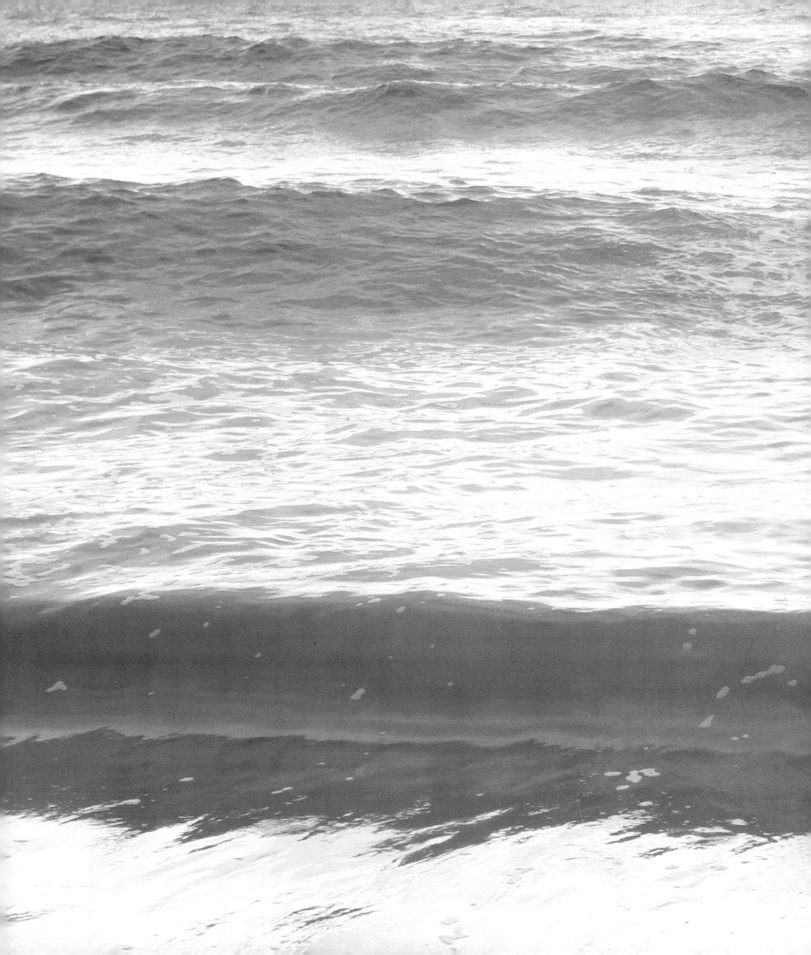

WATER

emotions, feelings, sensitivity, compassion, creativity, subconscious, perception

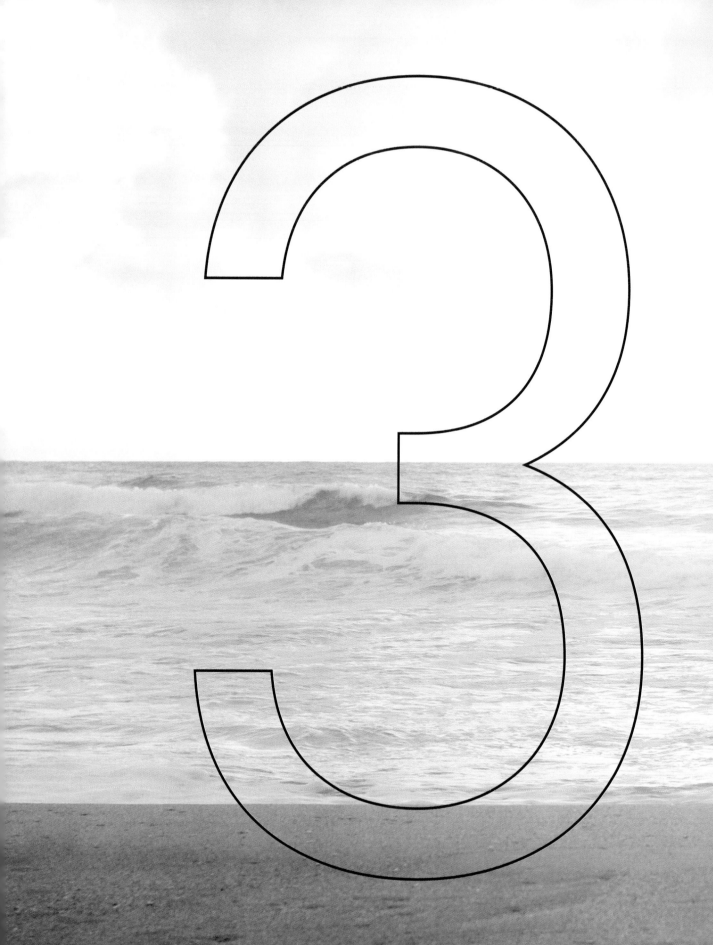

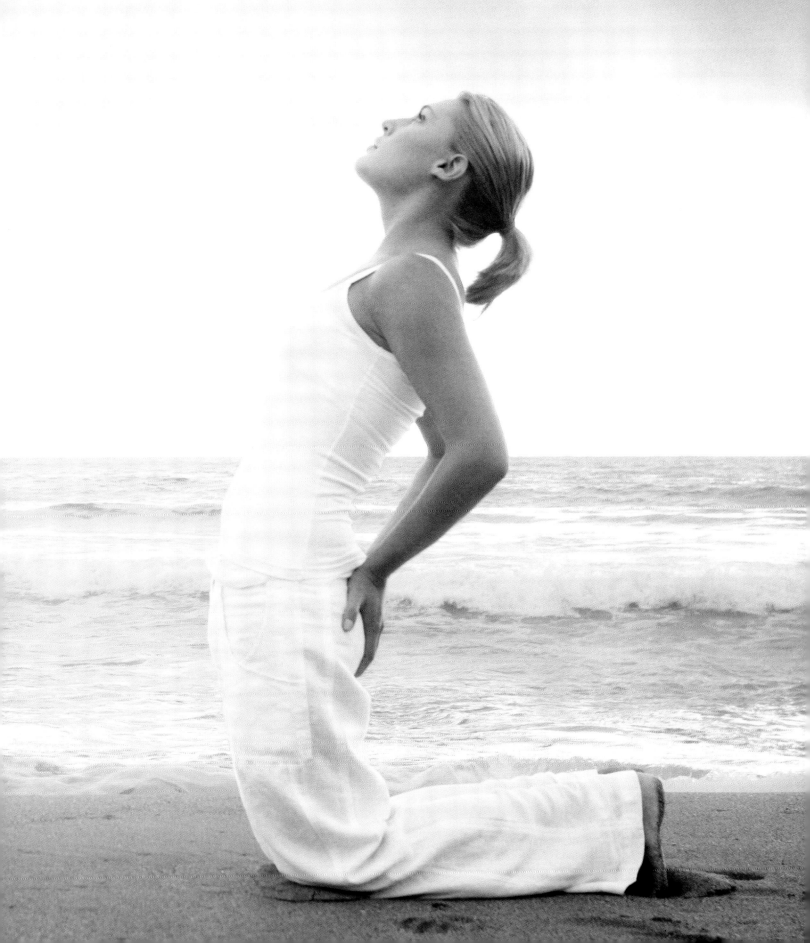

WATER The Kneeling Backbend represents the need to connect to our feelings and to the power of our subconscious mind. To do so gives us full access to our creativity.

As you practice this pose, you learn to become more like water, resisting nothing and simply flowing where it is easiest. You learn to feel the flow of your body in movement.

Take this awareness into your life—that resistance to change causes struggle. Learn to be more like water, adapting your shape (changing your perspective) to whatever contains you. Go with the flow, not against it. Areas of stagnation in your life are just areas where you have blocked the flow.

3RD RITE
THE KNEELING BACKBEND

Affirmation: "I am flexible and receptive."

INTRODUCTION

What lies behind us and what lies before us are small matters compared to what lies within us. Ralph Waldo Emerson

In yoga, backbends are known as expansive, extroverted movements that can elicit powerful emotional changes in your body and mind. Traditionally, they are undertaken toward the middle of a routine so that you have plenty of time both to prepare for them and to compensate after practicing them. The Third Rite—the Kneeling Backbend—maintains this integrity.

Like all of the Five Rites, the Kneeling Backbend is very powerful. It opens you up to life, awakening your vital energy, lifting your spirits and dispelling sluggishness. It is not unusual to feel a bit irritable or weepy after doing yoga, and in particular after carrying out backbends. As you spread open your chest, perhaps after years of it being collapsed and taut, you are in effect opening yourself up. Backbends can therefore be considered an excursion into the unknown, opening you up to feelings of vulnerability or insecurity, or even happiness! Give yourself time to experience feelings of joy, or to let go of tears or process anger, fear or other emotions. However, if you don't feel this release when practicing the backbend, don't feel that you are not doing the posture correctly. It is like most things in life: some people do, and some people don't. Everyone's experience is unique.

The Kneeling Backbend will make you more aware of the connection between your body and your mind. As you continue to practice the Rites, you loosen both your body and your mind. By overcoming your limitations physically or mentally, you are able to live a fuller life.

Benefits

According to the Tibetan lamas, this Rite influences the entire chakra system. It relieves muscular tension and opens out and stretches the muscles that shorten as your posture changes with age. These include the chest and shoulder muscles, and the muscles between the ribs and the front of the upper arms.

It lengthens and tones the entire spinal column, increasing spinal flexibility, particularly of the stiffest part of your spine—the thoracic region attached to your ribs. It helps to counteract the forward-bending change in the shape of our spine as we age. It opens up the pelvic area, massages the kidneys and lubricates the joints. It helps to dispel sluggishness and stagnation, stimulate digestion and regulate periods.

The Kneeling Backbend also stretches the whole of the front of the body, from the groin to the abdomen, to the chest and the throat. When your rib cage stretches you are able to breathe more deeply, which refreshes your whole body. As it opens the chest and the area around your heart, the stretch helps to dispel any heavy-hearted feelings.

PREPARATION

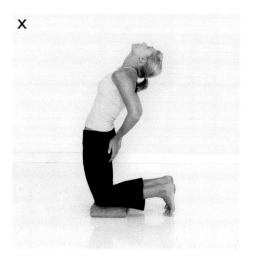

✗

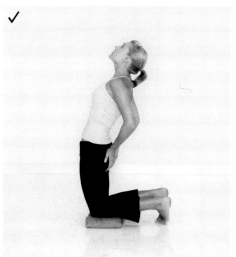

✓

1. **Caution**

   If you have any of the conditions listed in Part 1 on pages 20–21 or a history of disc or spinal injury, kidney disease, serious heart condition or high or low blood pressure, consult your doctor before attempting the Kneeling Backbend. If you have a history of knee, shoulder, back or neck injuries, it is advisable to consult a qualified medical professional before attempting this or any other posture. Avoid this Rite if you are pregnant, have a hernia or have had recent abdominal surgery.

   If you feel nausea or dizziness during the Rite, focus on opening your chest and shoulders rather than leaning back. Or do the exercise facing the back of a chair (see page 110)—further useful if you are unable to kneel on the floor.

2. **Equipment**

   If your floor is not carpeted or you need extra support for your knees, a small folded hand towel is ideal. (You may also require a second towel if you are unable to bend your toes; see page 110).

3. **"But I'm hardly moving"**

   Some people worry unnecessarily that they are barely moving in this movement. Never force a backbend—there should be no pressure on the lower back and it should be free of tension. Focus on stretching the thoracic area of your spine and opening your chest and shoulders.

4. **Lifting up out of your hips**

   You must practice and understand this concept before doing the movement.

   The goal is to create length between the hips and the ribs. This lengthening of the spine creates space between the vertebrae, helping to reduce pressure. You should aim to maintain this length throughout the movement.

   Sit upright on a chair with your feet flat on the floor. Tilt your chin down and focus your gaze on the middle of your chest. Place your hands on your hips with your thumb pointing backward. Inhale and start to lift your spine upward, and then lift your chest upward without overarching your back, and finally lift your head and look straight ahead. In other words, lift your ribs vertically away from your hips, without pushing your ribs forward.

5. **Keep your neck long and strong**

   When you move into the backbend, don't extend your head too far backward (see top left). It is crucial to hold the neck long and strong throughout this movement, to avoid occluding the vertebral artery, which would reduce blood flow and oxygen to the brain.

To keep the neck long and strong, think about stretching up through the crown of your head to the ceiling, and maintain this stretch when your head follows your back as you arch backward in the Kneeling Backbend (see opposite bottom).

6. **Counter stretch: Child's Pose**
After doing a backbend it is important to do a forward bend (a counter pose) to release any tension in your lower back and to bring your body back into balance. It is useful to learn this posture before you begin.

Exercise

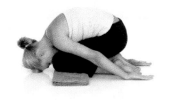

- Kneel on the floor, then sit back on your heels and fold your body forward, letting your forehead touch the floor. Your arms should be resting beside you with your hands toward your feet and your palms facing upward (see left). Note: If you are unable to touch the floor with your forehead, try resting it on one hand placed on top of the other. If that is still not enough height, make two fists with your hands and place them one on top of the other. Rest your forehead on the top fist.
- Allow your lower back to relax and stretch.

Warm-up
Cat Pose

This two-part stretch increases flexibility of the spine and helps you release any tension in your lower back before doing the backbend. Do not overextend.

Exercise

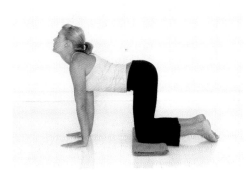

- Kneel on your hands and knees, with your hands directly underneath your shoulders and your knees directly underneath your hips.
- Engage your pelvic floor and pull your lower abdominals in toward your spine. Breathe out and let your back sag in the middle while looking upward (see left).

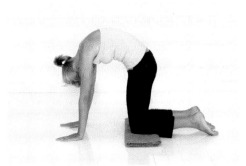

- Pause momentarily then, keeping your pelvic floor engaged, breathe in and arch your spine upward, tucking your chin into your chest (see left).
- Repeat the two-part stretch three times.

You are now ready to begin the Kneeling Backbend. If you find you need a little fine tuning along the way, turn to pages 110–111, for Solutions to Common Problems.

BEGINNERS

Remain at this level for week one of your practice, or until you are able to correctly perform the Rite. You will begin by doing three repetitions per day at this level.

For the first week you will do the Kneeling Backbend up close and facing a wall. The objective of this is to teach you how and where to extend your spine in this movement. Practice the posture in this manner until you are able to do it correctly. After week one and when you can maintain the movement, move on to the Intermediate/Advanced level.

Your aims

To master the technique of the Kneeling Backbend and to achieve three repetitions.

Instructions

1. Kneel with your knees close to the wall, hip-width apart and with your toes curled under. Your abdomen should be touching the wall. Check that your hips are positioned over your knees (move your knees back a bit if they are not). Don't thrust your pelvis forward. Wrap your hands under the cheeks of your buttocks.

    Breathing normally, lengthen your spine and lower your chin toward your chest. Make sure you are not hunching your shoulders toward your ears. This is the starting position.

    Lift your pelvic floor and pull your lower abdominals in toward your spine. Keep your focus on your lower abdomen and move from this central core throughout the movement.

    From here on, your breathing should be synchronized with the posture. Slowly inhale as you arch back into the posture, and slowly exhale as you return to your starting position (chin to chest).

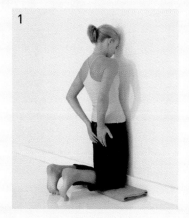 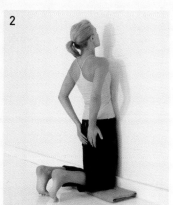 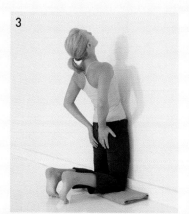 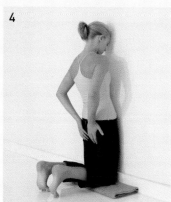

2. Gradually squeeze your buttocks firmly together and as you breathe in begin to lengthen your spine up and out of your hips. Press back against the foundation provided by your knees and legs to help you lengthen, then lift your breastbone upward. Keep your belly button pressed against the wall. If you are doing this step correctly, your stomach will "walk" up the wall a little way.

3. Stretch (do not force yourself) to a point of comfort then arch backward. As your spine arches, allow your head to follow, but do not let it collapse backward—keep your neck long and strong.

    Gently squeeze your shoulder blades together at the back and focus on opening your chest. Do not jerk the shoulders downward or thrust your chest up—do not force.

4. Breathe out slowly, keeping your pelvic floor engaged, and return smoothly and with control to your starting position (chin to chest).

5. Allow your muscles to relax. This completes one repetition.

6. Repeat this exercise for three repetitions.

7. When you have completed the Kneeling Backbend, move into the counter-stretch position (Child's Pose, see Preparation, page 105). Allow your lower back to relax and stretch out to compensate for the backbend you have just completed.

    Still in Child's Pose, move your knees slightly apart to prepare for Energy Breathing. As you breathe, focus on the muscles of your back—expanding and contracting. Begin by exhaling fully, then take three complete Energy Breaths ending on an inhalation (see page 35, Step One).

    To get up, place your hands on either side of your head and take a small breath, then use your hands to push yourself into an upright position, looking forward as you do so. Holding your breath until you come upright will reduce the possibility of you going red in the face or feeling a bit dizzy.

7

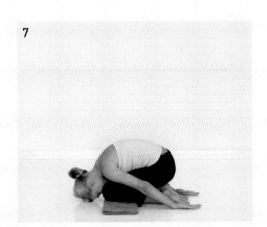

INTERMEDIATE/ADVANCED

Your aims

To take the technique learned at the Beginners level and perform it without the wall as a guide. Also to gradually build up to 21 repetitions.

Instructions

While you are still building up flexibility, do only a few stronger backbends and do the remainder of your repetitions less strongly.

1. Come into the starting position: kneeling on the floor with your toes curled under, your knees hip-width apart, your hips above your knees, your hands wrapped under the cheeks of your buttocks, and your chin lowered toward your chest. Make certain you are not hunching your shoulders toward your ears.

    Lift your pelvic floor and pull your lower abdominals in toward your spine. Keep your focus on your lower abdomen and move from this central core throughout the movement.

    From here on, your breathing should be synchronized with the posture. Slowly inhale as you arch back into the posture, and slowly exhale as you return to your starting position (chin to chest).

2. Gradually squeeze your buttocks firmly together and breathe in as you begin to lengthen your spine up and out of your hips. Press back against the foundation provided by your knees and legs to help you lengthen, then lift your breastbone upward (as if walking your abdomen up the wall).

3. Stretch (do not force yourself) to a point of comfort then arch backward. As your spine arches, allow your head to follow, but do not let it collapse backward—keep your neck long and strong.

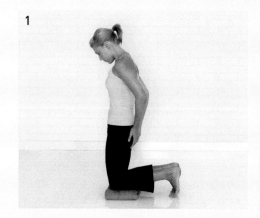
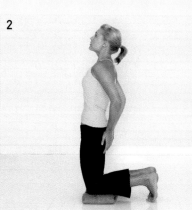
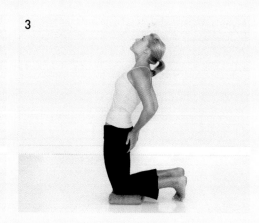

Gently squeeze your shoulder blades together and open your chest. Do not jerk the shoulders downward or thrust your chest up—do not force. You should feel this stretch in the thoracic (mid-back) region of your spine, as well as in your chest, shoulder and abdominal areas.

4. Breathe out slowly, keeping your pelvic floor engaged, and return smoothly and with control to your starting position (chin to chest).

5. Allow your muscles to relax. This completes one repetition.

6. Repeat the Kneeling Backbend in a steady, unbroken rhythm until you have completed your desired number of repetitions. Remember to add just two repetitions per week till you reach 21.

7. When you have completed the Kneeling Backbend, move into the counter-stretch position (Child's Pose, see Preparation, page 105). Allow your lower back to relax and stretch out to compensate for the backbend you have just completed.

   Still in Child's Pose, move your knees slightly apart to prepare for Energy Breathing. As you breathe, focus on the muscles of your back—expanding and contracting. Begin by exhaling fully, then take three complete Energy Breaths ending on an inhalation (see page 36, Step Two).

   To get up, place your hands on either side of your head and take a small breath, then use your hands to push yourself into an upright position. Holding your breath until you come upright will reduce the possibility of you going red in the face or feeling a bit dizzy.

4

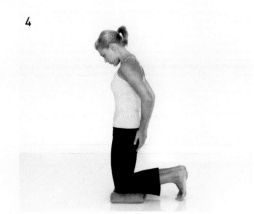

7

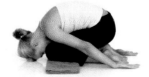

SOLUTIONS TO COMMON PROBLEMS

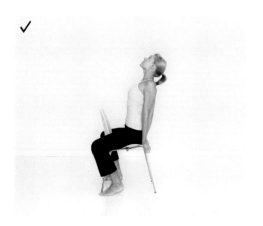

✓

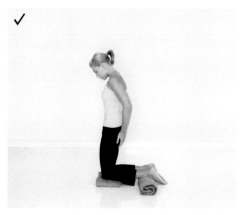

✓

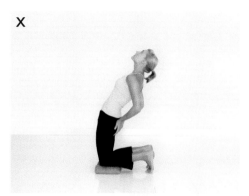

✗

1.   **Unable to kneel on the floor**
If you find kneeling uncomfortable, place a folded towel or blanket underneath your knees. If you are still unable to kneel on the floor for any reason use a chair instead (see left).

Sit facing the back of the chair. Place your feet on the floor and gently hold on to the base of the chair with your hands for support. Follow the instructions for the Kneeling Backbend.

2.   **Unable to bend your toes**
If your toes are too stiff to curl under in the kneeling position, try using a pillow, blanket or folded towels to support and hold your feet in position (see left) while you perform this Rite.

To increase flexibility in your toes, interlace your fingers between your toes and rotate them, stretch them and generally move them around to reduce stiffness. Another useful exercise is to come into the kneeling position, tuck your toes under as best you can, then slowly lower your bottom onto the back of your calves, giving your toes a good but comfortable stretch. Aim to eventually sit on the backs of your legs. Do this latter stretch whenever you can: a good time is while you are watching television.

3.   **Overbending in your lower back**
To avoid overextending (collapsing) your lumbar area in the Kneeling Backbend, you are taught to stabilize your hips and lower back with your buttocks and core stability muscles. This prevents any movement of the hips so that you have a strong foundation from which to lean backward. In the Kneeling Backbend, the aim is not to collapse in the lower back as you lean backward, but to focus on opening your chest and creating length between your hips and the stiffest part of your back, the thoracic spine. If you haven't completed exercise 4 (page 104) in Preparation, do so now.

4.   **Leaning back on your thighs**
Your hips and thighs should remain stationary throughout the movement in this Rite. They act as an anchor for you to push back against as you stretch up and backward. If you find you are leaning back on your thighs (see left), place your hands on your hip bones to remind you to keep your hips and thighs still.

X

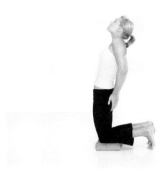

5. **Hunched shoulders**

Some people attempt to lengthen their spine by lifting their shoulders toward their ears (see left). By practicing "walking the abdomen up the wall" (see Beginners, pages 106–107), you will learn how to extend your spine correctly. Once you have lengthened your spine, be very mindful to let your shoulders rotate down and back, then gradually squeeze your shoulder blades together at the back.

6. **Lack of control**

Move slowly and cautiously throughout this movement; do not jerk or make sudden, sharp movements. Some people arch back smoothly, but when it comes to returning to their starting position, they suddenly let go. This is rather like stretching a rubber band as far as it will go, and then releasing it instantly! Avoid any sudden collapsing of your spine by returning to your starting position in a smooth and controlled manner, keeping your spine elongated.

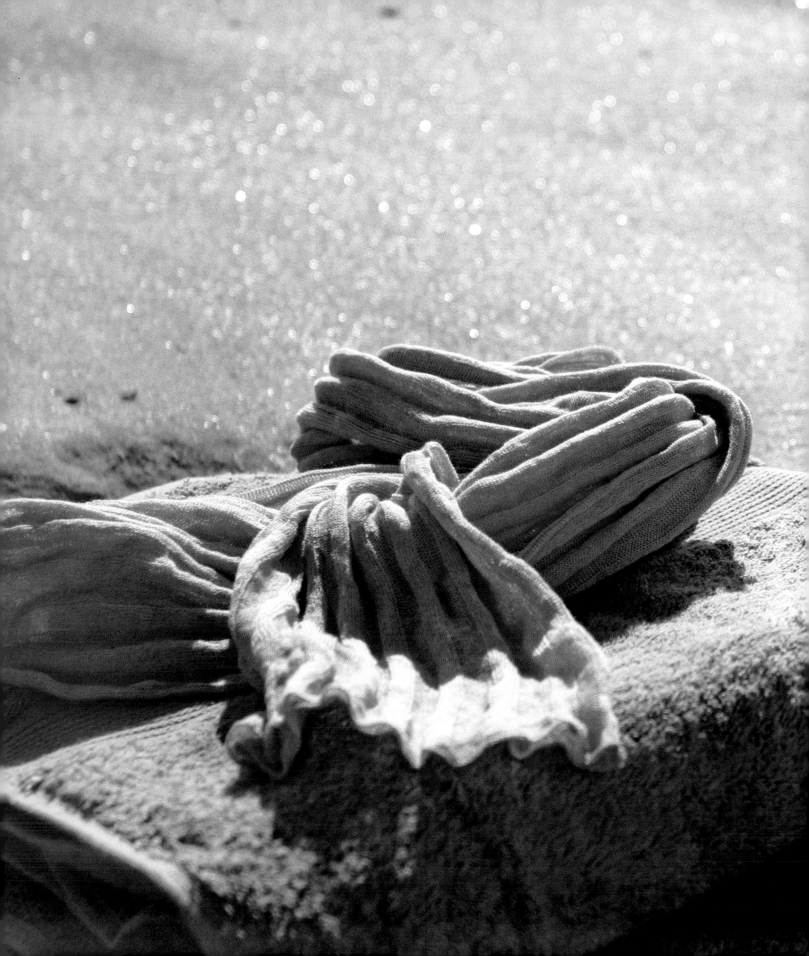

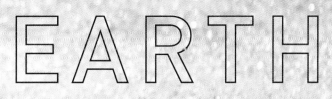

EARTH

*stability, self-discipline,
ambition, solidity,
productivity,
nurturing, order*

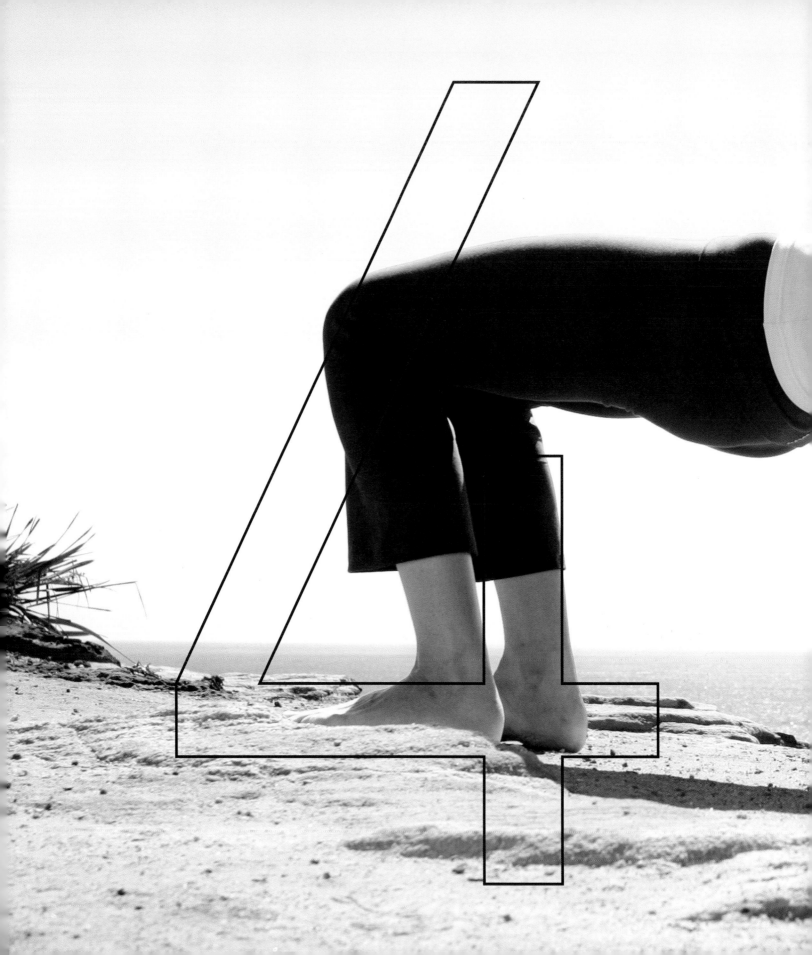

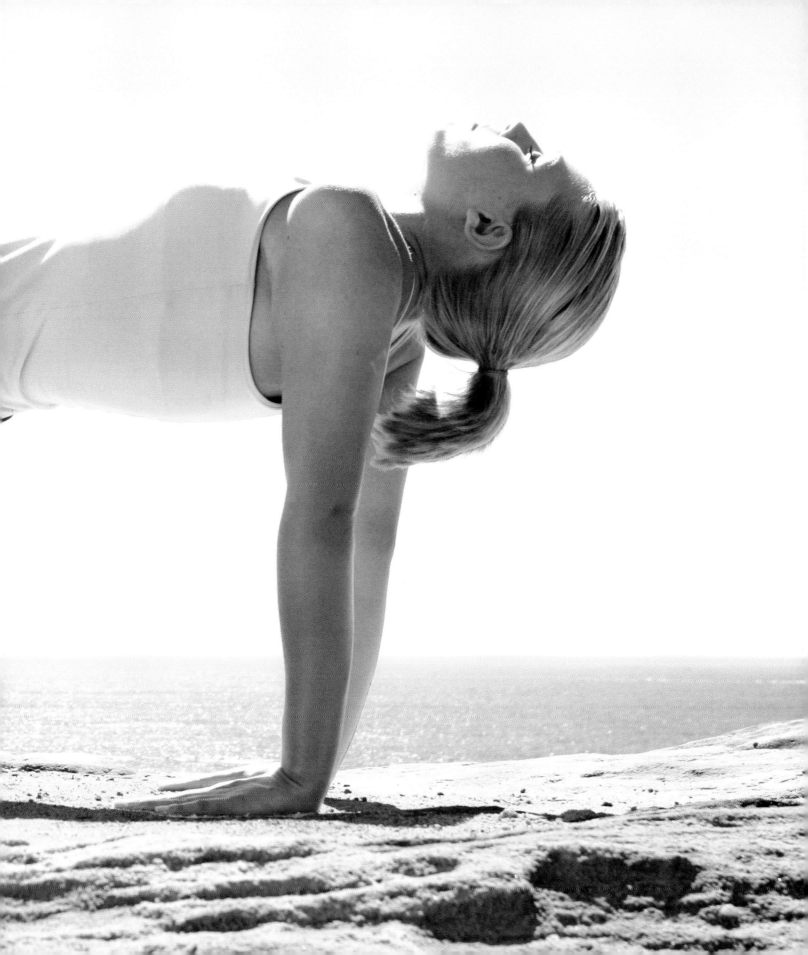

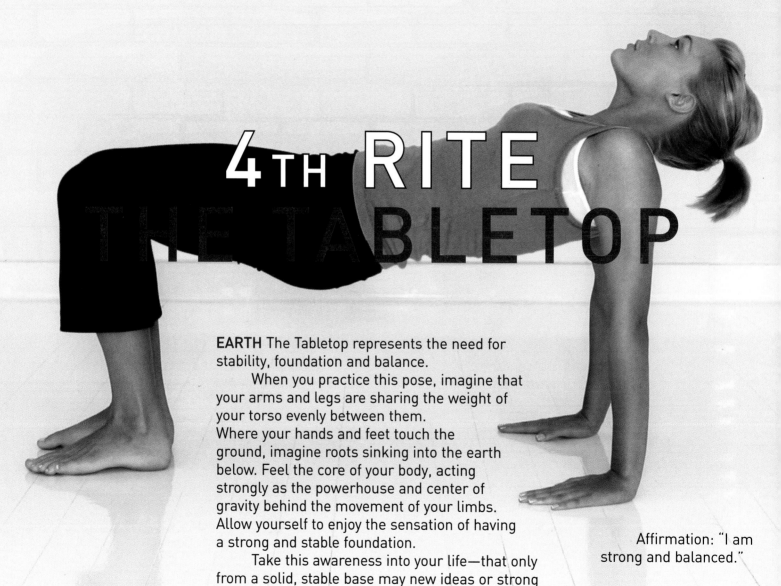

4TH RITE
THE TABLETOP

EARTH The Tabletop represents the need for stability, foundation and balance.

When you practice this pose, imagine that your arms and legs are sharing the weight of your torso evenly between them. Where your hands and feet touch the ground, imagine roots sinking into the earth below. Feel the core of your body, acting strongly as the powerhouse and center of gravity behind the movement of your limbs. Allow yourself to enjoy the sensation of having a strong and stable foundation.

Take this awareness into your life—that only from a solid, stable base may new ideas or strong relationships (professional or intimate) be brought successfully into form.

Affirmation: "I am strong and balanced."

INTRODUCTION

I am always doing things I can't do, that's how I get to do them.
Pablo Picasso

The Tabletop looks harder than it is. In my workshops, my students are always delighted and somewhat surprised to discover how much easier this posture is than they had imagined. It is all a matter of learning the tricks.

When you haven't used your body for quite a while, you lose "connection" with it to some degree. It takes a while to gain confidence in using muscles that haven't been active for some time. For this reason the Tabletop is taught in progressive stages. Don't push yourself at any stage; it's neither necessary nor desirable.

The Tabletop is a balancing and weight-bearing posture. It is true that your balancing skills diminish with age, but the good news is that poor balance is not inevitable. Balance-recovery strategies can be very effective, no matter what your age, and both the Spin and the Tabletop are helpful in improving balance.

Benefits

The lamas claim that this Rite stimulates the minor chakras in the knees, and the major chakras from the reproductive centers to the throat.

The Tabletop is an effective but safe weight-bearing exercise. By performing it you will develop strong arms, wrists and shoulders. In many people's experience, arms that had become loose and flabby become toned and attractive again. The Tabletop is also very good for strengthening your knees, thighs, hips, back and lower abdominals.

The Tabletop helps improve your balance by assisting you to find and work with, and therefore better understand, your center of gravity (your core).

It is also great for stretching and opening out your chest, helping you to breathe more deeply.

Finally, but important, the Tabletop stimulates your nervous, circulatory and lymphatic systems, and boosts your vitality.

PREPARATION

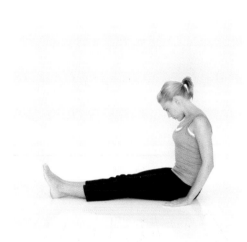

1. **Caution**

   If you have weak wrists or abdominal muscles, weakness or stiffness in the shoulders or legs, lower back pain or neck pain, progress slowly with the Tabletop, adding only one or two repetitions each week. If you have any of the conditions listed in Part 1, pages 20–21, gain your doctor's approval before attempting this posture.

2. **Finding correct sitting position**

   The correct sitting position (see left) is the starting position for this Rite.

Exercise

- Sit upright with your legs in front of you, shoulder-width apart. Make sure your body is resting on your two sitting bones and keep your knees soft and unlocked. If you don't know where your sitting bones are, place your hands underneath your buttocks: you will feel them protruding.

- Place your hands by your sides, with fingers pointing toward your toes. Lengthen your spine by pushing back against your sitting bones. Imagine there is a cord running from the crown of your head to the ceiling, pulling you upright.

- Without arching your back or puffing your ribs outward, lift your breastbone upward, and open your chest.

- Drop your chin toward your chest so that the muscles at the back of your neck remain long and strong.

- Slightly bend your arms and rotate the creases of your elbows slightly forward toward your feet. This will help you keep your shoulder blades back and down.

You are now in the correct starting position: your back is straight, your chest is open, your arms are by your sides with the elbows rotated slightly forward, and your chin is on your chest.

   In the early stages you may not have the strength to sit with your back upright while you figure out what to do next. This is fine—while you are getting yourself into the correct starting position, sit however you like, but the moment you are ready to move into the posture, straighten your back, then put your chin on your chest. If you begin in a hunched-over position, you will lose the leverage of the movement that helps you get into the Tabletop position. Losing this leverage makes it much harder to achieve.

3. **Correct arm and shoulder position**

In the starting position, draw your shoulders away from your ears as you lengthen your spine.

Rotating the crease of your elbows slightly forward has the effect of rotating your upper arms backward, expanding the chest and broadening the back. This assists the muscles of your upper back to engage more effectively when lifting into the Tabletop.

During the first few lifts, some people may need to turn their hands out to the sides slightly. This is fine: for some people, having their hands out to the sides increases their comfort level but still allows their shoulders to rotate back and down. However, aim to eventually have your fingers pointing forward.

4. **Finding correct hand position**

Everyone has different-sized arms and legs, so you will need to find the hand position that is most comfortable for you.

When you first try this posture, place the balls of your palms next to the top of your thighs. (You may need to adjust this.) Place your palms on the floor with the fingers pointing toward your toes. Spread your fingers a little, pressing each knuckle evenly onto the floor. This will ensure that the weight of your body is distributed evenly across your whole hand.

Generally, shorter-armed people need to place their hands further forward and longer-armed people need to place them further back. The only way to find out is to try it. Remember that the goal is to be evenly weighted in the lift between legs and arms. Two methods of finding the best position for you are outlined in the section on achieving equal balance between your arms and feet (see page 120).

a) Short arms or weak wrists

If you notice that your arms feel uncomfortably short in this exercise, you may need to place something firm like folded towels or wooden or foam blocks under the palms of both hands to get the height you need.

If your arm or wrist strength is weak, blocks will make it easier to elevate and prevent you from jerking.

Try the following adaptations first, but for a more permanent solution, wrist and arm strengthening exercises are given on page 130.

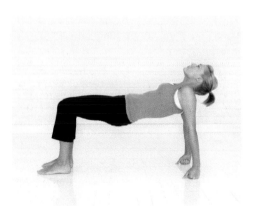

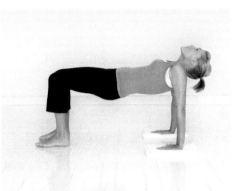

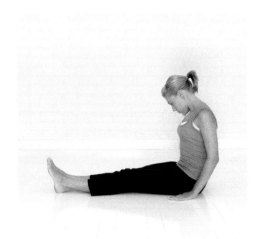

Doing the posture on your knuckles
Form your hands into fists with the fingers facing inward. Doing the posture on your knuckles (see left) takes the strain off your wrists. Over time, work toward doing the posture with your palms on the floor.

Using a towel
Fold a couple of hand towels into thick bands. Place your hands on the middle of the towels (see left). The towels will help elevate your arms, to balance them with your legs.

b)   Long arms
If you have long arms, try placing your arms further back at the start (toward your buttocks, away from your thighs) by about ½ inch.

5.   **Achieving equal balance between arms and feet**
a)   Method 1
If you lift into the Tabletop position and feel that most of your weight is on your shoulders, come back down and move your hands a little, either backward or forward. Then try the lift again, coming back down and adjusting your hands until you find the right spot. You may find that as little as a quarter of an inch can make all the difference to you being balanced in the lift. When you come back down into the starting position, make a mental and visual note as to exactly where your correct hand position is.

   Note: In the Tabletop posture, your feet should be in full contact with the floor. If they aren't—for example, if your toes are sticking up—your feet are not taking the full weight they should and you will be placing most of your weight on your shoulders. If this is the case, follow the instructions in Method 2 below.

b)   Method 2
Another way of finding your point of balance is to imagine you are a plank of wood when you are in the Tabletop position. Simply slide your body toward your feet a little and then back a bit, until you find the point at which it is most balanced. When you get it right you will know, because it feels comfortable. This is only a small movement, yet it can make a great difference to your comfort. Make certain all ten toes are in full contact with the floor.

6.   **Focus on your lower abdomen to lift**
As you lift into the Tabletop and let yourself down again, make certain you lift your pelvic floor and pull your lower abdominals in toward your spine. Keep your focus on your lower abdomen and move from this central core throughout the movement. Apart from protecting your spine, this helps you to keep your body aligned and not moving from side to side.

7.   **Use your legs to drive your knees over your ankles**

Once you have lifted your bottom off the floor, use your legs to drive your knees up and toward your toes, placing all ten toes in contact with the floor and your knees over your ankles. This will help you get into the Tabletop position with the minimum amount of strain, by using the stronger muscles of your legs instead of your arms.

If your middle is still sagging, it is possible you are starting with your arms too far forward. In your starting position, place your hands a few centimeters backward and try it again. This should lengthen your tabletop and allow your trunk to form a straight line between your feet and your hands. If this does not work, you need to develop more strength in your pelvis and buttocks. Your daily practice of the Tabletop will help you achieve this but if you require more help, try the strengthening exercise for weak pelvis and buttocks on page 131.

8.   **How long should you hold the Tabletop position?**

With a long, slow inhalation "breathe" (lift) yourself up into the Tabletop position. Tense briefly at the top of your lift, then exhale slowly as you lower yourself back down into the starting position.

You are now ready to begin the Tabletop. If you find you need a little fine tuning along the way, turn to pages 128–129 for Solutions to Common Problems.

BEGINNERS/INTERMEDIATE/ADVANCED

STEP ONE

There is only one level of this Rite (Beginner/Intermediate/Advanced) but it is learned in three steps. The reason they are steps (and not levels) is because there is no need to remain at each of the steps for any set length of time; as soon as you have achieved the goals of each, you can move straight on to the next.

Step One of the Tabletop involves sliding your bottom along the floor to your heels, and back again. Perform this step several times until you are able to achieve all the aims below. At this point you can move straight on to Step Two—there is no need to remain at Step One for any set period of time or number of repetitions.

Note: If you have a tiled or timber floor it will make it easier for you to slide your bottom toward your heels. If you find this step too uncomfortable, go straight to Step Two.

Your aims

To be able to slide your bottom toward your heels and back to your starting position without moving the position of your feet or hands. And to flatten your feet and all ten toes onto the floor, so that your weight is evenly distributed across each foot.

Instructions

1. Come into the correct starting position: sitting on the floor with your back straight, your breastbone lifted, your chin to your chest, and the creases of your elbows rotated forward (see Preparation, page 118).
    Unlock your knees.
    Lift your pelvic floor and pull your lower abdominals in toward your spine. Keep your focus on your lower abdomen and move from this central core throughout the movement.

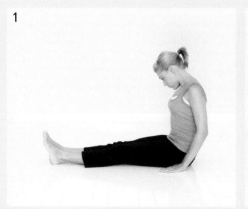
1

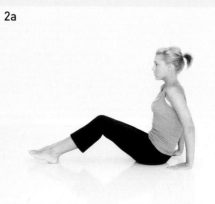
2a

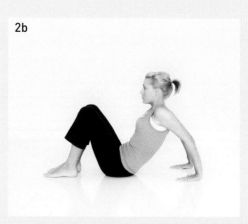
2b

2.   Breathe in and at the same time slide your bottom toward your heels. Focus on flattening your feet and all ten toes onto the floor.

3.   Keeping your pelvic floor engaged, breathe out as you slide your bottom back to the starting position, where your hands are next to the tops of your thighs.

4.   Repeat this action several times until you are comfortable and can achieve all the aims of Step One.

If you are able to achieve the aims of Step One, progress to Step Two immediately. Otherwise, remain at Step One until you can achieve it easily. Refer to the strengthening exercises on pages 130–131, if necessary.

5.   If you are remaining at this level until your strength has built up, lie down with your knees bent and place your hands in the Energy Breathing Position with your hands wrapped around your lower ribs.
      Exhale fully, then take three complete Energy Breaths ending on an inhalation (see pages 35–36, Steps, One, Two and Three).

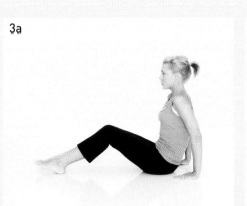

3a

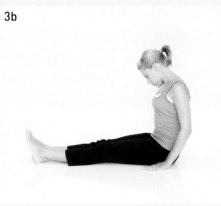

3b

STEP **TWO**

Step Two involves lifting your bottom slightly, moving it toward your heels and placing your feet flat on the floor, then moving your bottom back again. Perform this step several times until you are able to achieve all the aims below. As with Step One, when you are able to perform Step Two you can move straight on to Step Three—there is no need to remain at Step Two for any set period of time or number of repetitions.

Your aims

To be able to lift your bottom slightly from the correct sitting position, then move it toward your heels, without pulling your legs back toward you. And to make certain that you bring your buttocks right back to your starting position with the heels of your palms next to the tops of your thighs and your legs straight.

Instructions

1. Come into the correct starting position: sitting on the floor with your back straight, your breastbone lifted, your chin to your chest and the creases of your elbows rotated forward (see Preparation, page 118).

    Unlock your knees.

    Lift your pelvic floor and pull your lower abdominals in toward your spine. Keep your focus on your lower abdomen and move from this central core throughout the movement.

2. Breathe in and at the same time lift your bottom slightly off the floor and use your legs to drive your knees forward toward your toes, coming to rest above your ankles. Don't worry about lifting your pelvis upward, just attempt to flatten your feet and all ten toes onto the floor.

1
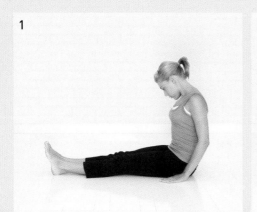

2a
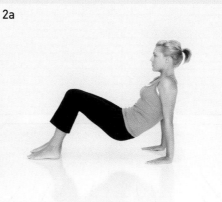

2b
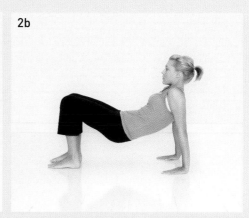

3. Keeping your pelvic floor engaged, breathe out as you move your bottom (which will remain slightly elevated) all the way back to your starting position, where your hands are next to the tops of your thighs.

4. Do this step several times, until you are able to get your feet straight and flat on the floor, and then your buttocks all the way back to the starting position.

If your arms or wrists are still weak, remain at this step until strength has built up. Once you have achieved the aims above, progress to Step Three immediately.

5. If you are remaining at this level until your strength has built up, lie down with your knees bent and place your hands in the Energy Breathing Position with your hands wrapped around your lower ribs.

Exhale fully, then take three complete Energy Breaths ending on an inhalation (see pages 35–36, Steps One, Two and Three).

3a

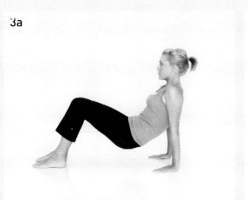

3b

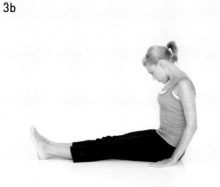

STEP THREE

Step Three takes you into the full Tabletop position.

Your aims

To lift cleanly into the Tabletop position, synchronizing your breathing with the movement. To be able to flatten all ten toes onto the floor and to move in and out of the posture without shifting the starting position of the arms and legs. To build gradually up to 21 repetitions.

Instructions

1. Come into the correct starting position: sitting on the floor with your back straight, your breastbone lifted, your chin to your chest and the creases of your elbows rotated forward (see Preparation, page 118).

    Unlock your knees.

    Lift your pelvic floor and pull your lower abdominals in toward your spine. Keep your focus on your lower abdomen and move from this central core throughout the movement.

2. Breathe in and lift your bottom off the floor, then use your legs to drive your knees up and forward toward your toes, coming to rest above your ankles. At the same time, let your head and shoulders move backward toward the floor behind you. Do not jerk from the arms—this is more of a rolling action onto the balls of your feet, with a simultaneous smooth curling backward of the head.

    Concentrate on getting the soles of your feet, and all ten toes, on the floor, and raise the middle of your abdomen and chest into a straight line (tabletop) above the floor, with your arms straight. Do not let your head hang backward.

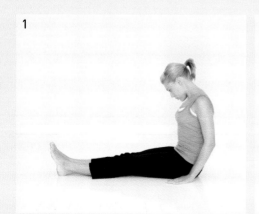
1

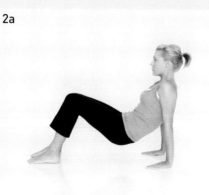
2a

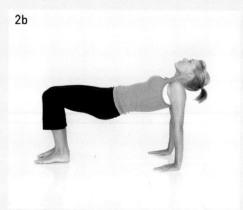
2b

Keep it long and strong, in the same position as it would be when standing, or with your chin lightly tucked against your chest. If you prefer, you can hold your head upright.

You will now look like a tabletop: knees bent, feet on the floor, stomach and chest in a straight line above the floor, straight arms, and your neck long and strong. Do not push your stomach so far upward that you bend in the middle of your lower back. Once in this position, tense your muscles briefly.

3. Check that your pelvic floor is lifted and your lower abdominals are pulled in, then breathe out while focusing on your lower abdominal muscles to guide your body back into your starting position. As you come back down, make certain you keep moving your bottom back toward your arms until your legs are totally straight.

4. Relax your muscles in the starting position. This completes one repetition.

5. Each time you begin the Rite, straighten up first and make sure your chin is to your chest.

Repeat the Tabletop in a steady, unbroken rhythm until you have completed your desired number of repetitions. Remember to add just two repetitions per week until you reach 21.

6. Lie down with your knees bent and place your hands in the Energy Breathing Position with your hands wrapped around your lower ribs.

Exhale fully, then take three complete Energy Breaths ending on an inhalation (see pages 35–36, Steps One, Two and Three).

3a

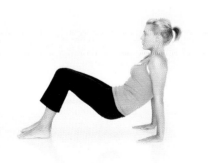

3b

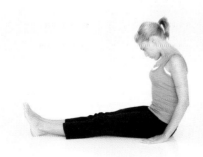

SOLUTIONS TO COMMON PROBLEMS

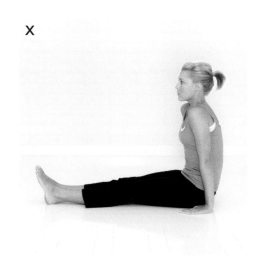

X

1. **Feet together**

   The aim of this posture is to balance your weight equally between your arms and your legs. A common tendency is for people to lift with their feet together, forming a three-legged table. This does not distribute weight evenly across the body and is very unstable—your legs should be shoulder-width apart. As you perform the Tabletop, literally imagine yourself as a well-balanced table.

2. **Unable to straighten legs**

   If you are unable to straighten your legs in front of you in the starting position, aim to do so over time. It simply means you have tight leg muscles, which will become more flexible as you practice T5T.

3. **Locking knees and elbows**

   Some people lock their knees before they lift their pelvis off the ground at the beginning of the movement. To avoid strain on the knee joints, keep your knees soft. To lift, use the muscles of the thighs and buttocks instead of the knees.

   A number of people lock their elbows, too, often when psyching themselves up to use their arms to lift their body off the ground. This action causes strain and creates a sharp, jerky movement. Keep the elbow joints soft and rotated forward at the beginning of the movement. If you can't lift yourself into the Tabletop position at first, don't worry: give your muscles time to strengthen.

4. **Hunching to start**

   When you come back down into the starting position, your body may be slightly hunched forward (see left). This is normal, but make sure you straighten up before each repetition. Doing this gives you the best leverage potential for your next lift, making it easier to achieve and avoiding injury.

   Note: When you tip your chin to your chest in the starting position, make certain it is just a small tuck of the chin toward the chest. Some people exaggerate it so much that they cause their shoulders to hunch over.

5. **Moving feet**

   In this Rite your feet do not move position, they simply flatten onto the floor and then come back up. Some people have a tendency to slide their feet back along the floor toward their buttocks to help them do the posture. Make certain your heels stay in the same position all the way through the Tabletop.

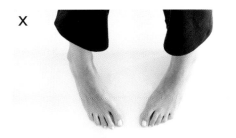

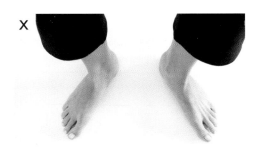

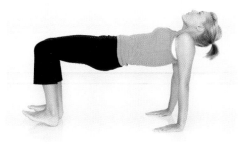

6. **Incorrect feet**

Placing your feet in a pigeon- (see top left) or duck-toed (see middle left) position puts strain on your joints. Aim for your feet to be straight in line with your body. If your toes are sticking up (see bottom left), it is an indication that your weight is uneven. Aim to put all ten toes in direct contact with the floor, so that the weight of your torso is evenly distributed between both feet as well as between your arms and your legs.

7. **Moving across the floor**

If you are doing the Tabletop correctly, your starting and finishing position will be exactly the same. If you find yourself moving across the floor you will be doing one of two things. First, check that you are not pulling your feet toward you, as in Moving Feet (opposite). Second, check that you are bringing your buttocks *all the way* back to your starting position. Some people come back only part of the way and then have to move their hands forward to line up with the tops of their thighs again.

FURTHER TIPS

If you are currently lacking in strength, it is very important to understand that you *will* be able to do this Rite if you allow yourself time. People with weak wrists, shoulders or legs or with a weak abdomen will find the following strengthening exercises helpful.

Do the exercises listed here daily until you have built up enough strength to perform the beginning steps of the Tabletop easily. As you practice these steps, you will continue to naturally develop strength in the shoulders and arms, readying you for the full version of the Tabletop. It is simply a matter of practice and time.

1. **Weak wrists**

   If your wrists are lacking in strength or are tight, you may need to perform the following exercises daily for a few weeks to build up your strength. Do only the number of repetitions you can perform comfortably and without strain.

   a) Ball squeeze

   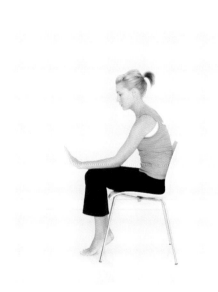

   Place a soft rubber or tennis ball in the middle of the palm of your hand and squeeze the ball 15 to 20 times (or more if you are able).

   b) Wrist lifts

   In the sitting position, place the length of your right forearm along the length of your right thigh with your hand hanging over your knee, palm downward. Keep your forearm on your thigh and move your hand up (see left) and down from the wrist as many times as you are able to do comfortably.

   Now flip your palm so it is facing upward, and do the same up-and-down movement. Swap hands and repeat both movements. As your strength increases, hold ordinary household objects in your hands as weights.

   c) Wrist stretch

   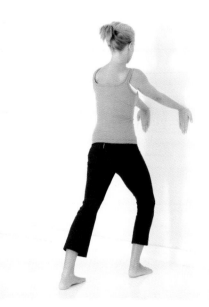

   Stand facing a wall. Place your hands side by side in front of you with your palms upright as if someone was about to give you something. Tip your fingers down toward the ground and place your palms against the wall. Slide one leg behind you while bending the other knee (see left). Press your hands firmly against the wall, so that you can really feel the stretch in your wrists. Hold the stretch for a count of five, or less if it becomes uncomfortable, then relax. Repeat several times.

2. **Weak shoulders or arms**

   Daily practice of the steps of the Tabletop will naturally strengthen your arms and shoulders. When you find it easy to achieve each step, simply move on to the next.

3. Weak pelvis and buttocks

If you find it hard to get your bottom off the floor, rest assured you are not alone. Further good news is that if you just follow the steps, in time you will be able to do it. In many ways this gradual achievement will be more motivating for you than being able to do it straightaway.

If you do have difficulty in lifting your pelvis upward, you may need to teach your muscles a new trick. Alternatively, it may be a case of incorrect technique, muscle weakness or lack of confidence. Try correcting your technique first. Otherwise be patient and allow your strength to build with time. The following exercise will help you to develop strength in your pelvis, buttocks and legs.

a)   Strengthen your pelvis

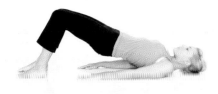

Lie on your back with your knees bent and your arms by your sides, palms down. Lift your pelvic floor and pull in your lower abdominals. Breathe in and at the same time slowly lift your pelvis off the floor as high as you can go (see left). At the top of the lift, tense your muscles momentarily. Check that your pelvic floor and lower abdominals are engaged and then breathe out while slowly lowering your pelvis back to the floor.

Gradually build up to 10 repetitions of this strength-building exercise, until you are able to lift your pelvis fully into the air, making a straight line with your body.

4. Weak thighs

Once again, your daily practice of any of the steps in the Tabletop will naturally help you to develop strength in your legs. When you find it easy to achieve one of the steps, simply move on to the next. The following strength-developing exercises are also useful.

a)   Leg holds

Sit on a chair with both feet on the floor. Straighten your right leg and hold it there for 5 to 10 seconds. Return your foot to the floor. Repeat 5 to 10 times with your right leg, then swap legs and perform the same number of repetitions. Aim to practice leg holds three times a day.

b)   Calf lifts

Do this exercise next to a wall, so that you can place your hand against it if you need to stabilize yourself. Stand with your feet hip-width apart. Lift your pelvic floor and pull your lower abdominals in toward your spine for balance. As you breathe in, raise both of your heels off the floor, so that you are standing on the balls of your feet. Without pausing, breathe out and slowly let your heels come back to the floor. Repeat this "pumping" action 5 to 10 times: breathe in and lift, breathe out and down.

FIRE

*intuition, insight, new ideas,
heat, passion, willpower, confidence,
strength, expansion, and the dual
nature of fire—destruction
and creation*

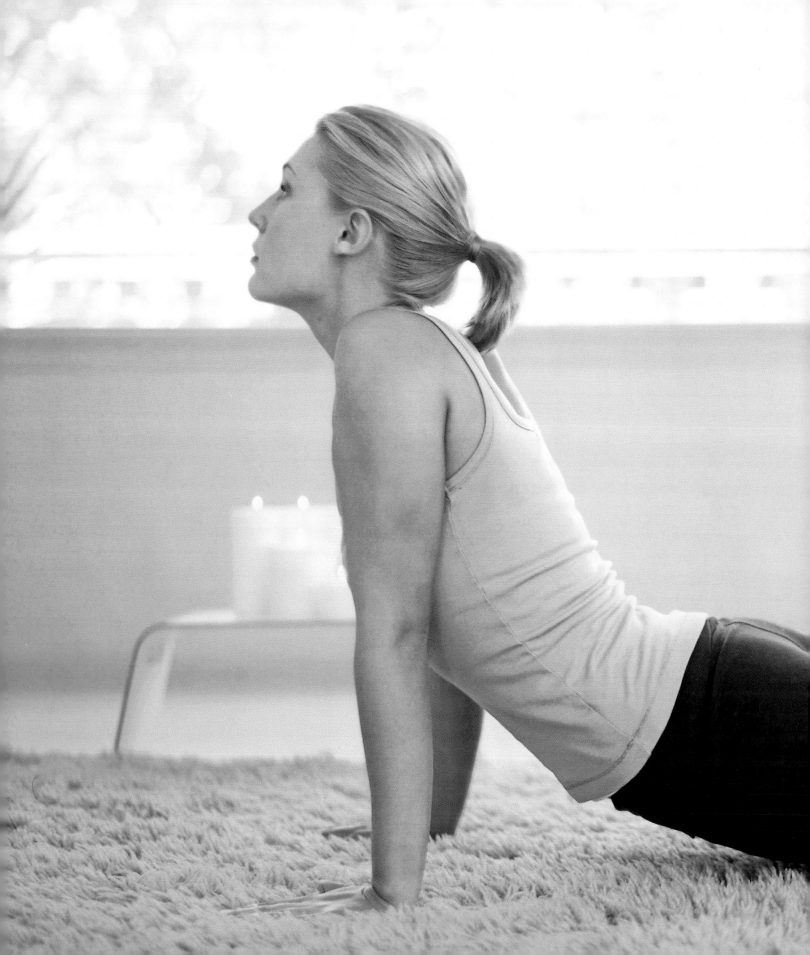

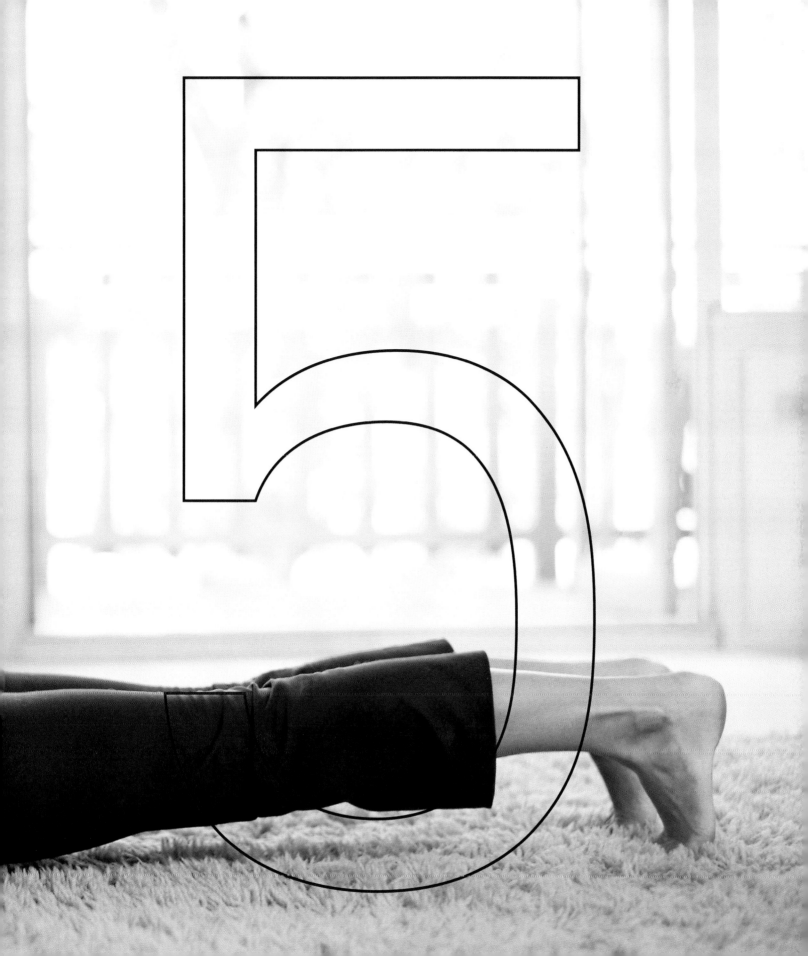

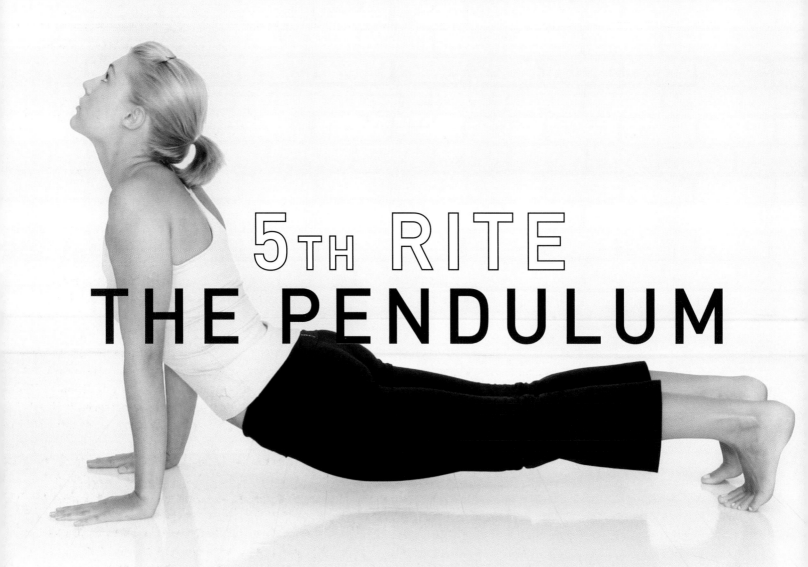

5TH RITE
THE PENDULUM

FIRE This pose represents the need for energy, motivation and courage to follow one's intuition. It symbolizes the need to destroy old ways of thinking so that one can expand and create new ways of being.

When you practice this pose, imagine that the in–out pump-like action of the movement is recharging you with energy and vitality and dispelling sluggishness and negativity.

Take this awareness—that you have within you the ability to "destroy" what you don't want in your life and to "create" what you intuitively seek—into your normal life. When you carry out these two actions with awareness and deliberation, you will have the motivation, strength and confidence to bring new ventures into being.

Affirmation: "I am positive and motivated."

INTRODUCTION

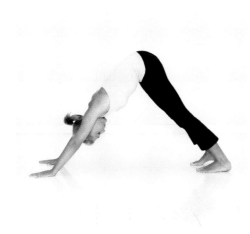

What you get by achieving your goals is not as important as what you become by achieving your goals.
Johann Wolfgang von Goethe

The final posture in T5T is a powerful energizer and eliminator. Like the other four before it, this Rite has a stimulating effect upon the human energy system. When done together, the Five Rites have a cooperative effect that results in the stimulation of all the chakras of the body, creating a healthier and a more physically, emotionally and spiritually balanced person.

The upside-down V shape or downward-facing dog position is one of the most familiar yoga poses and provides a very rejuvenating stretch for most of the body. The Fifth Rite begins with downward-facing dog and ends with a modified version of upward-facing dog. These two traditional yoga postures flow from one into the other and represent a dog stretching after waking from a nap.

I named this Rite for its backward-and-forward swinging motion, like that of a pendulum.

Benefits

This dynamic Rite works most of your body.

The two parts of the pose combine to produce a powerful stretch that can be felt from your tailbone to the top of your neck, as your whole spinal column elongates and opens, freeing tension. It is a very invigorating and refreshing exercise that fills you with energy.

It is brilliant for improving flexibility. In downward dog, you open out the entire back of your body with an intense stretch to the back of your legs, including your calves and ankles. Holding your head in the downward position relaxes your face, throat and neck. Upward dog concentrates on opening up the entire *front* of your body, with an intense stretch to your abdomen and chest. By performing the Pendulum, stiffness in your back, legs, hips and shoulders is relieved and continues to reduce over time.

The Pendulum strengthens your spine, back, shoulders, arms, wrists and legs, and firms your buttocks! By building muscle and increasing flexibility it improves your posture. The weight-bearing nature of the pose also stimulates your bones to retain calcium.

The Pendulum stimulates your nervous system and improves your circulation. It increases blood flow to your head and opens up your chest, allowing deeper breathing. It can also assist with sinus congestion. The increased oxygen and *prana* give you more energy and vitality. Most of your major organs are also stimulated in the Fifth Rite, as are your lymphatic, hormonal, digestive and eliminative systems. It stimulates your abdominal organs and may reduce sluggish or irregular periods, and bowel or digestive disorders.

As you build up repetitions, the dynamic nature of the Pendulum shifts mild depression and relieves fatigue and stress. The dual nature of the pose both calms and energizes you.

PREPARATION

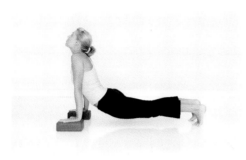

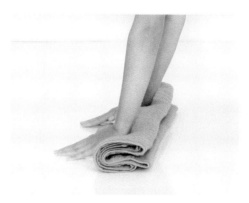

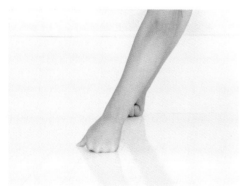

1. **Caution**

    Avoid this exercise if you have uncontrolled high blood pressure, carpal tunnel syndrome, glaucoma, retinal injuries, wrist or back injury or are pregnant. It is advised not to perform this posture if you have a headache or diarrhea. If you have any of the conditions listed in Part 1 on pages 20–21, gain your doctor's approval before attempting the Pendulum.

2. **Weak wrists**

    If your wrists are initially quite weak, the suggestions below might make things easier while you develop strength. They will also help if you are having trouble with the posture due to stiffness. Remember to take as many rests as needed.

    a) Yoga blocks

    Giving yourself some height by placing your hands on yoga blocks places more weight onto your legs in downward-facing dog and takes pressure off your wrists. Also it makes it easier for you to remain elevated above the floor in upward-facing dog (see top left).

    b) Towels or yoga mat

    If you find the yoga blocks too high, try using a towel (or yoga mat) folded to about five centimeters (two inches) thick. Place your palms toward the furthest edge of the towel so your fingers can touch the floor (see left). Lower the height of the towel as strength or flexibility increases.

    c) Knuckles

    Alternatively you can do the Rite on your knuckles (see left). Form a fist with each hand, with your thumb curled outside your fingers. Place your hands on the floor as shown.

3. **Keeping the movement straight**

    Find a vertical line in the carpet markings or timber joins (or stick down a straight line of tape), and position yourself with the line running along the middle of your body. Due to differences in strength between the left and right sides of our body, some people incorrectly skew the movement to one side. If you favor your stronger side all the time, you will not develop strength on the other side. Skewing to one side can also put pressure on the joints. Move your body along the "middle line" during the movement to avoid this imbalance.

4. **Starting position**

    The starting position for the Pendulum is on your hands and knees with a "middle line" along the center of your body and your back straight.

    Place your knees directly below your hips and your hands a little wider than shoulder width. Now move your hands farther forward by about five centimeters (two inches). Spread your fingers so that your weight is evenly distributed across your whole hand. Make sure your legs and arms are level.

5.   **Support your lower back**
     In Step Three, as you start to descend from downward-facing dog in order to swing through your arms into upward-facing dog, make sure you lift your pelvic floor and pull your lower abdominals in toward your spine. Smoothly squeeze your buttocks together and hold this contraction all the way up into upward-facing dog—at the end of the movement your buttocks should be firm but not hard. Using your core stability muscles in combination with squeezing your buttocks ensures that you control the speed and degree by which you lower your lumbar spine during the transition. This protects your lower back.

Finishing
Child's Pose

It is lovely to complete the full sequence of the Rites with a posture of relaxation. This calming moment allows all the energy that is rushing around in your body to settle. It gives you time to stretch, relax and recover for a few minutes, and to prepare for the remainder of your day. (If Child's Pose is too uncomfortable, simply roll over onto your back and lie there with your knees bent for a few moments.)

Exercise

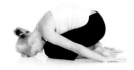

- From your hands and knees, slowly lower your bottom toward your heels.
- Fold your body forward, letting your forehead touch the floor. Your arms should be resting beside you with your hands toward your feet and your palms facing upward (see left). Note: If you are unable to touch the floor with your forehead, try resting it on one hand placed on top of the other. If that is still not enough height, make two fists with your hands and place them one on top of the other. Rest your forehead on the top fist.
- Breathe normally for a few moments.
- To get up, place your hands on either side of your head, take a small breath and then use your hands to push yourself into an upright position. Holding your breath until you come upright will reduce the possibility of you going red in the face or feeling a bit dizzy.
- From the kneeling position, place one bent leg in front of you and overlap both hands over the knee. Push on the knee with your hands to lift your body upward and over the knee into the standing position.

You are now ready to begin the Pendulum. If you find you need a little fine tuning along the way, turn to pages 146–148, for Solutions to Common Problems.

BEGINNERS/INTERMEDIATE/ADVANCED

STEP ONE

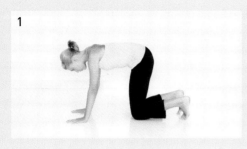

1

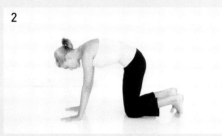

2

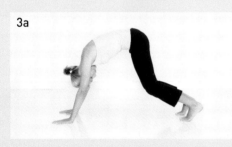

3a

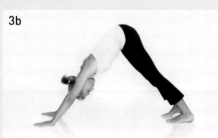

3b

The Pendulum is learned in steps instead of levels. This is because the three steps are different parts of the same movement. First you learn how to perform downward-facing dog, second you learn upward-facing dog, then, at Step Three, you link the two poses with a transitional movement.

If you are familiar with and able to perform downward-facing dog and upward-facing dog, you can go straight to Step Three.

Do Step One of the Fifth Rite until you are confident of the steps. Some people will want to stay at this level until their arm and leg strength increases, while others will do it once and move straight on to Step Two.

Your aims
To correctly perform downward-facing dog—then coming back down onto bent knees, and moving up again into downward-facing dog. To synchronize your breathing with the movement.

Instructions
1. Come into the starting position (see Preparation, page 138) and make sure that your back is straight.

2. Spread your fingers out and attempt to distribute your weight across your whole hand, including the fingers.
    Rotate the creases of your elbows slightly forward. Spread and curl your toes under.
    Lift your pelvic floor and pull your lower abdominals in toward your spine. Keep your focus on your lower abdomen and move from this central core throughout the movement.

3. Breathe in and continue to inhale as you move your head downward toward your chest, lifting your knees off the floor and pushing your hips up and back— bringing your body into an upside-down V shape with your tailbone pointing toward the sky.
    Make sure your arms are fully extended, with your shoulder blades drawn back and down toward your tailbone.
    Tilt your chin toward your chest, relax your neck and look at your feet. Your back should be flat, not rounded—you will probably need to work toward achieving this over time.
    Relax the back of your legs and ankles and allow your heels to drop toward the floor as best you can. Straighten your legs as much as you can but don't lock your knees.

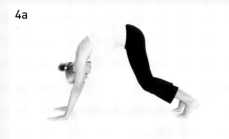

4a

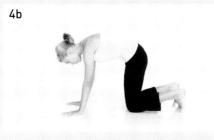

4b

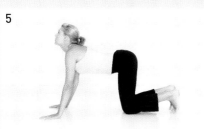

5

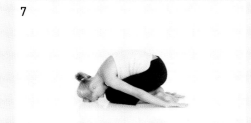

7

Lift your buttocks and tailbone up toward the ceiling.
Attempt to distribute your weight evenly between your arms and legs.

4.   Breathing out, bend your knees back down to the floor.

5.   On your hands and knees, gently hollow the middle of your back so that your tailbone points up in the air. Your back will be arched upward a bit and your head will move gently backward. This completes one repetition.

6.   Engage your pelvic floor and pull your lower abdomen in toward your spine before moving into the next repetition as follows: breathe in and continue to inhale as you press back against the balls of your feet and come back into the upside-down V shape.

7.   If you are able to achieve the aims of this step, move straight to Step Two. If you wish to remain at this level until your strength and flexibility improve, finish now by coming into Child's Pose (see Preparation, page 139) for a few moments of relaxation, or carry out one of the two breathing exercises in Part 4, pages 153–156.

STEP **TWO**

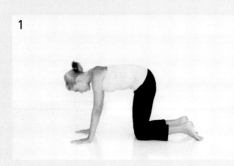

1

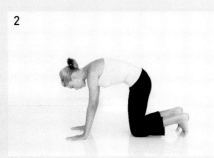

2

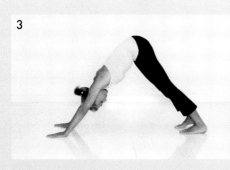

3

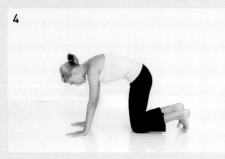

4

When you have mastered Step One you are ready to add the second part of the posture—upward-facing dog.

When you are able to achieve the aims of this posture easily and without strain, you are ready to move on to Step Three.

Your aims

To learn the second part of the Pendulum—upward-facing dog. To synchronize your breathing with both downward-facing dog and upward-facing dog. To keep your buttocks firmed while you elevate your legs off the floor. To keep your body weight distributed evenly between your toes and hands.

Instructions

1. Come into the starting position (see Preparation, page 138) and make sure that your back is straight.

2. Spread your fingers out and attempt to distribute your weight across your whole hand, including the fingers.

   Rotate the creases of your elbows slightly forward. Spread and curl your toes under.

   Lift your pelvic floor and pull your lower abdominals in toward your spine. Keep your focus on your lower abdomen and move from this central core throughout the movement.

3. Breathe in and continue to inhale as you push down through your toes, lifting your knees off the floor and pushing your hips up and back—bringing your body into an upside-down V shape with your tailbone pointing toward the sky.

   Make sure your arms are fully extended, with your shoulder blades drawn back and down toward your tailbone.

   Tilt your chin toward your chest, relax your neck and look at your feet. Your back should be flat, not rounded—you will probably need to work toward achieving this over time.

   Relax the back of your legs and ankles and allow your heels to drop toward the floor as best you can. Straighten your legs as much as you can but don't lock your knees.

   Lift your buttocks and tailbone up toward the ceiling.

   Attempt to distribute your weight evenly between your arms and legs.

4. Breathing out, bend your knees back down to the floor.

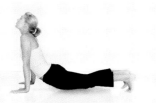

5. Breathe normally, squeeze your buttocks and engage your lower abdominals and spread your legs out straight behind you (or take small steps backward). Shift your weight forward over your wrists. Your knees should be in contact with the ground.

    Squeeze your buttocks and look up, letting your back and head arch gently backward, and your shoulders descend away from your ears. You are now in a modified version of upward-facing dog.

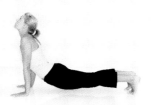

6. When you feel strong and steady, still squeezing your buttocks firmly together and keeping your lower abdominals engaged, lift your knees and legs off the ground by pressing down through your toes. Stretch out through your heels to straighten your legs. You are now in the full version of upward-facing dog. This completes one repetition.

7. Breathe out and keeping your lower abdominals engaged move your tailbone into the downward-facing dog position; and so on to complete your desired number of repetitions.

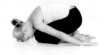

8. If you are able to achieve the aims of this step, move straight to Step Three. If you wish to remain at this level until your strength and flexibility improve, finish now by coming into Child's Pose (see Preparation, page 139) for a few moments of relaxation, or carry out one of the two breathing exercises in Part 4, pages 153–156.

STEP THREE

When you have mastered downward-facing dog and upward-facing dog, you are ready to learn the correct transition movement that smoothly links the two postures.

Your aims

To be able to control the lowering of your body in the transitional movement, through the use of your core stability muscles and squeezing of your buttocks—to ensure that your lumbar spine is kept stable without collapsing. To be able to carry out this movement with straight arms.

Instructions

1. Come into the starting position (see Preparation, page 138) and make sure that your back is straight.

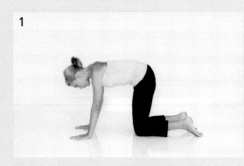

2. Spread your fingers out and attempt to distribute your weight across your whole hand, including the fingers.

    Rotate the creases of your elbows slightly forward. Spread and curl your toes under.

    Lift your pelvic floor and pull your lower abdominals in toward your spine. Keep your focus on your lower abdomen and move from this central core throughout the movement.

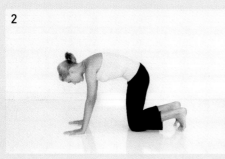

3. Breathe in and continue to inhale as you push down through your toes, lifting your knees off the floor and pushing your hips up and back—bringing your body into an upside-down V shape with your tailbone pointing toward the sky. Make sure your arms are fully extended with your shoulder blades back and down toward your tailbone.

    Tilt your chin toward your chest, relax your neck and look at your feet. Your back should be flat, not rounded—you will probably need to work toward achieving this over time.

    Relax the back of your legs and ankles and allow your heels to drop toward the floor as best you can. Straighten your legs as much as you can but don't lock your knees.

    Lift your buttocks and tailbone up toward the ceiling.

    Attempt to distribute your weight evenly between your arms and legs.

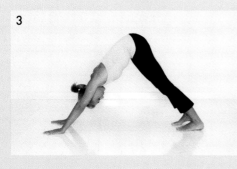

4. Engage your pelvic floor and lower abdominals. Breathing out, start to move your head and upper body down and through your arms, keeping them *straight* at all times with the creases of your elbows slightly rotated forward.

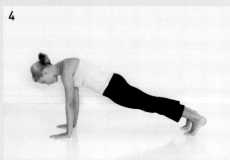

5

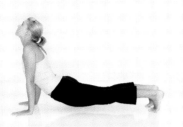

8

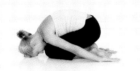

5. Keep your pelvic floor and lower abdominals engaged and gradually squeeze your buttocks firmly together to support your lower back, as you come up into the full upward-facing dog position. Draw your shoulders away from your ears, and lift your breastbone upward without puffing out your ribs. Aim for length rather than height.

    Make sure your pelvis and legs are not touching the floor—only your hands and curled-under toes should be in contact with the floor. Push your heels backward to prevent you coming up onto your tiptoes. This is the full stretch.

6. Repeat these movements for the desired number of repetitions in a smooth, flowing and continuous action—almost like a pendulum. You should be breathing in as you move up, and out as you move down.

7. When you have finished your repetitions, simply bend your knees and drop them to the floor so that you are back on your hands and knees.

8. Come into Child's Pose (page 139) for a few moments of relaxation, or carry out one of the two breathing exercises in Part 4, pages 153–156.

SOLUTIONS TO COMMON PROBLEMS

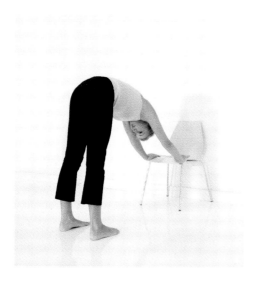

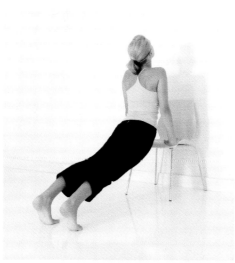

1. Very stiff

If you are very stiff, it might be useful to begin with an easier version of the Pendulum. Place a sturdy and level chair against a wall; the back of the chair should be against the wall. Stand in front of the chair and place your hands shoulder-width apart on the front edge of the chair. Prepare for downward-facing dog by taking a large step backward, until you are a full arm's length away: take another little step backward if necessary. Lift your pelvic floor and bring your lower abdominals in toward your spine. Breathe in, then push against the chair and raise your tailbone, lengthening your spine and stretching from your fingertips to your bottom bones (see left).

For upward-facing dog, firmly grip the seat of the chair and with your buttocks squeezed and your lower abdominals engaged, bring your pubic bone and the tops of your thighs toward the chair. Keep your arms straight, with your shoulders rolled back. Focus on lengthening your spine by lifting up your breastbone and opening out your chest (see bottom left). Avoid collapsing your lower back.

To come out of the posture, return to the downward dog position and walk your feet toward the chair, then stand up slowly.

2. Downward-facing dog

a) Rounded back

To lengthen and straighten your back requires a fair degree of flexibility and strength. Be patient! Focus on lifting your tailbone toward the ceiling. Lengthen your spine by stretching your pelvis away from your hands. Draw your shoulder blades back and down toward your tailbone and imagine a straight line running from the tip of your middle finger, up your arms and back, to your sitting bones.

b) Heels can't touch the floor

It is not uncommon for people to be unable to put their heels on the floor. Work toward being able to do this over time. Note that in this pose your body should be equally supported by your arms and legs; as well as moving your heels toward the floor, aim to extend your arms fully and draw your shoulder blades down and back toward your tailbone. Focus on keeping your back straight and lifting your tailbone toward the ceiling.

c) Slipping feet

Not everybody's feet slip but if yours do, perform the posture with the back of your heels against a wall.

d) Strain on the back of your legs

If you feel strain on the back of your legs, slightly bend your knees. Work at straightening them over time.

e) Too much pressure on the arms
Focus on shifting your weight back onto your legs to help relieve pressure on your arms. Alternatively, use yoga blocks as suggested in Preparation (see page 138).

3. Transition
Transition is the movement down from downward dog into upward-facing dog.

a) Feeling "stuck"
When moving from downward-facing dog into upward-facing dog, some people feel a bit "stuck short"—like they can't move any farther forward. The easiest way of solving this is to walk your feet back an inch or so until you can easily perform the transition into upward-facing dog.

b) Bent arms
Keep your arms completely straight throughout the movement, particularly as you swing down from downward-facing dog and up into upward-facing dog. If you bend your elbows at this stage you will have to perform a very strong push up. This isn't correct or desirable.

c) Tense shoulders
Beginners often tense their shoulders in the transition by pulling them up toward their ears. As you swing through your straight and firm arms, rotate the soft part of your elbow forward and actively draw your shoulder blades down toward your tailbone.

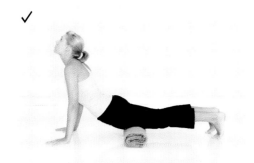

d) Difficulty in elevating legs off the floor or weakness in the lower back
In the beginning stages, you may find it easier to support your thighs in upward-facing dog. Place a rolled-up thick towel or firm pillow horizontally between your knees and hands in the starting position. When you come down from downward-facing dog and start to move into upward-facing dog, the towel will cushion and support your weight in the mid region of your thighs (see left). As your strength develops, aim to remove this support so that your legs are suspended above the floor and your whole body weight is supported at either end by your hands and toes. Caution: do not get so comfortable on your support that you collapse your lower back. To protect your lower back from sagging, make sure you firm your buttocks and enlist the support of your core stability muscles.

4. Upward-facing dog
a) Lifting too high
To avoid strain in your lower back, aim for length in the spine rather than height. Don't let your lower back sag by ensuring that your pelvic floor is lifted,

your lower abdominals are pulled in toward your spine and your buttocks are firmly squeezed. (If you tip your head back, take care not to compress the back of your neck.)

If you feel any discomfort in your lower back, don't lift so high and look straight ahead instead. Again, aim for length rather than height, and keep your head, neck and shoulders relaxed to avoid strain. Draw your shoulder blades away from your ears. Lift your breastbone up without puffing out your ribs, which has the effect of lengthening your spine as opposed to arching it. You may find it easier to learn this movement by using yoga blocks, as outlined in Preparation on page 138, or a support under your thighs.

b)   Balancing on your tiptoes

If you are on the tips of your toes in this pose, you will feel like you are about to topple over. Press back firmly against the balls of your feet to establish good contact with the floor. (Pushing your heels backward is a good way to achieve this.) As your feet press more firmly against the floor you will feel much more stable and it will be easier to lengthen your body and lift your breastbone up and forward as required.

Congratulations! You've now learned the Five Rites!

Over time, as awareness of each posture develops, I am sure you will discover, as I did, that the Five Rites are a masterfully blended dance of energy.

I remember one gentleman watching a few of us demonstrate the full sequence. When we had finished he had a wonderful look of calm and peace all over his face and he said in genuine amazement, "That was beautiful." Indeed it is!

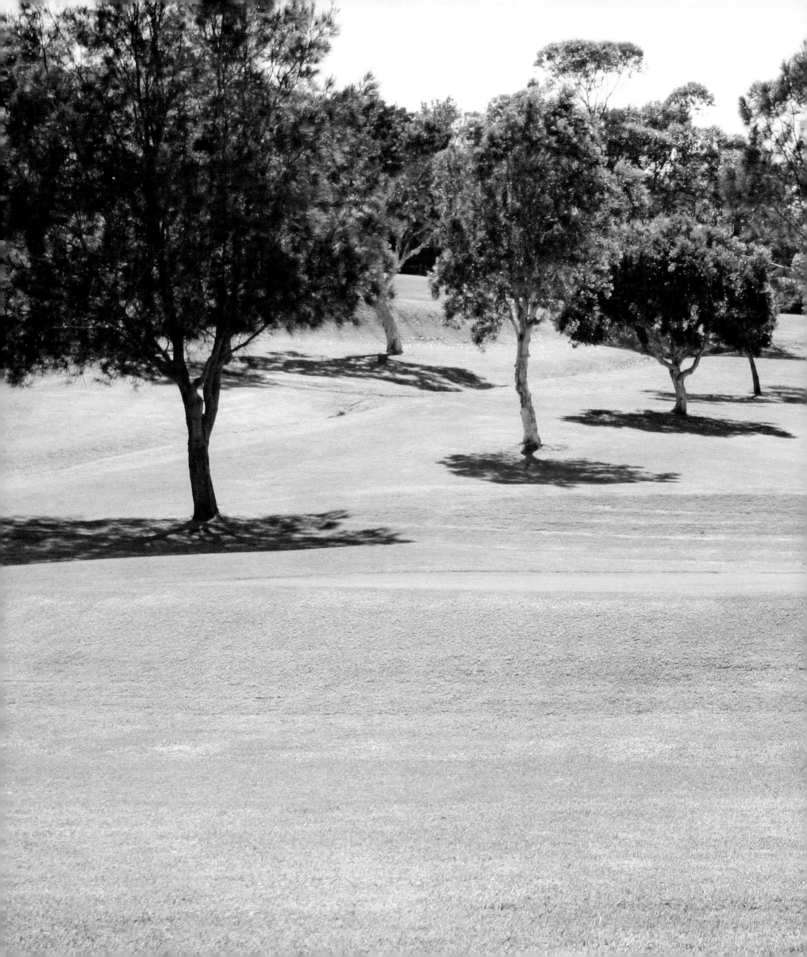

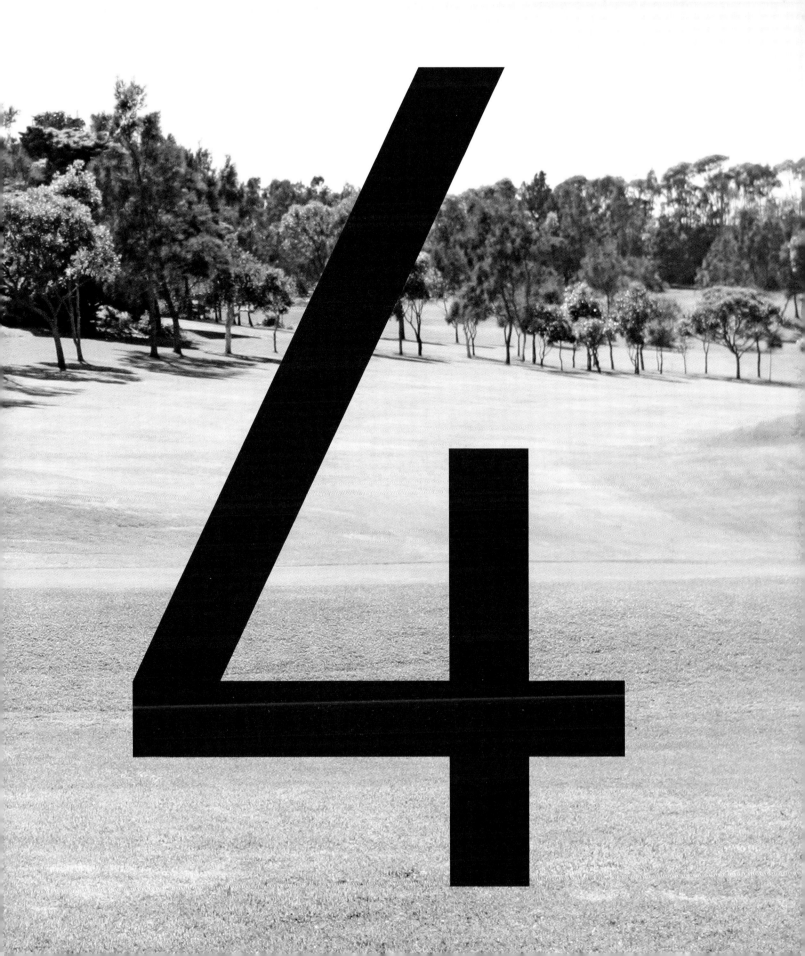

As for the proper inner breath, it is called the embryonic breath. Since it is naturally inside you, you do not have to see outside for it. Master Great Nothing of Sung-Shan, from the Taoist Canon on Breathing

In our modern world there seems to be a never-ending need for things to move faster and faster, toward some future event. We find it hard to relax and to experience the present moment. Finding time to experience the peace in silence has become something we have to schedule into our lives.

If you even remotely believe, as the ancients did, that we have only a finite number of breaths before we expire, then spending those breaths wisely will not only prolong your life, it will improve the quality of your life.

The following two breathing techniques replace the stress response with the relaxation response. They are wonderfully calming and even profound.

THE ONE BREATH

The One Breath is a simple and potentially profound relaxation and stress-management technique.

It is a very useful exercise for when you don't have much time and want to harmonize your mind, body and spirit. It is also an excellent way to end your T5T practice, helping you establish a sense of peace for the remainder of your day.

This exercise is equally effective for brief as well as extended periods of time, including meditation, and can also assist you in going to sleep.

The breath is easily taken for granted, yet it is profound. The air on this planet is constantly recycled and all living things share this air, breathing in nutrients and breathing out wastes. When we are born, we take our first breath of this communal earth air, and when we die we return our last breath back to the earth. Having this awareness before you begin this exercise can help you relax and trust the breath more deeply.

While you sleep your breathing is automatic, almost as if "you are being breathed." During this exercise you are going to become conscious of the breath, but you are going to try to maintain the perception that *there is nothing you have to do, except allow yourself to be breathed.*

Your aims

To initiate the relaxation response and to experience the fullness of your breath without the usual day-to-day restrictions.

Instructions

- Sit or lie in a comfortable position with your eyes closed.

- Bring your attention to your breathing and just observe it without trying to control it in any way.

- Now relax further and simply observe (witness) the natural ebb and flow of the breath being breathed into you and then withdrawn from you. Notice how and where the breath moves you: how your spine lowers and lifts and how your head rolls slightly forward and backward.

- As you feel the breath being breathed into you, imagine this life-enhancing breath entering your body and permeating every single cell, from the tips of your toes to the tip of your nose.

- As the breath is withdrawn from you, imagine all the wastes of your body flowing toward your lungs and then leaving with the out-breath.

- Surrender yourself to the feeling of being breathed for a few minutes. If your mind wanders, simply bring your awareness back to this exercise and continue.

- Notice how your breathing has slowed and deepened as you no longer attempt to control it. It is almost as if a deep, slow, natural breath has always been with you.

- When you are ready, begin to breathe normally once more. Allow yourself a few moments to reorient yourself before getting up and moving, calm and alert, into your day.

THE ENERGIZING AND HEALING BREATH

This second breathing exercise, the Energizing and Healing Breath, is included for those who wish to perform a deeper healing and reenergizing of their body. It can be practiced for extended periods of time as a relaxation or stress-control technique, or to assist you in falling asleep.

You can either memorize the steps or record them and play them back to yourself as you perform the exercise.

A beneficial exercise at any time, The Energizing and Healing Breath is particularly useful after your T5T practice. Focus on those areas that felt stiff, tense, weak or imbalanced as you carried out the Rites. This breathing technique utilizes the power of visualization to assist in healing these "stuck" areas and provides a wonderful feeling of well-being and calm that will last throughout your day.

Your aims

To utilize the power of visualization to rejuvenate and enrich your body with nutrient-rich oxygen and *prana*—and to remove wastes. To relax, restoring new energy and vitality to your body, mind and soul.

Instructions

- Lie or sit comfortably, so that no aches or discomfort will disturb your attention. If lying, have your knees bent with your feet on the floor and your arms by your sides. If sitting, have your legs slightly apart, your arms resting in your lap.

- Relax, and allow your weight to surrender you to the floor or the chair. If sitting, make certain that your back is straight and your shoulders are relaxed.

- Close your eyes, relax your face and jaw and begin to breathe in and out through your nose.

- Focus your awareness on the gentle ebb and flow of your breathing.

- Now begin to double or simply extend your exhalation.

- Establish the rhythm of breath that is most fluid, smooth and relaxing for your body, while continuing to double or extend your exhalation time.

- As you inhale, visualize fresh oxygen moving throughout your body, energizing each and every cell. As you exhale, visualize the carbon dioxide and other wastes moving out of your body.

- Bring your attention to your nose, where the air is entering your body. Imagine the oxygen and life force swirling down through your nasal passages and throat and swirling into and around your lungs. Tell yourself that with every breath you take in, healing energy is swirling into your body.

- Now imagine the carbon dioxide and wastes in your exhalation, as it moves back up and out of your body, taking with it any tension, discomfort, pain or illness.

- Bring your awareness now to your abdomen. Imagine a pair of nostrils in the middle of your belly through which you are now breathing. Visualize the oxygen coming in and swirling all around your abdomen, bowel, inner organs and lower back, bringing healing energy with it. Imagine the oxygen and life force penetrating deep into areas of darkness or stagnation, refreshing you and healing you.

- As you exhale through the imaginary nostrils in your belly, visualize any tension, pain or negative feelings flowing up and out of your body to be released.

- Now visualize a pair of nostrils in the center of your chest, near your heart, through which you are now breathing. Imagine the oxygen and life force swirling all around your chest, your ribs, your shoulders and your back, delivering oxygen and healing energy.

- As you exhale through the imaginary nostrils near your heart, imagine all the stress, negative emotions and anxiety leaving your body.

- Now bring your awareness to a part of your body that is tense, tired, or in some discomfort or pain.

- Visualize a pair of nostrils located right in the middle of this point. Imagine the oxygen and life force entering the nostrils and swirling all around the area of tension, pain or discomfort. With each inhalation, healing energy is swirling in and permeating every cell in that area. With each exhalation, tensions, pain or impurities are taken away, leaving that part of your body refreshed, cleansed and healed.

- Continue this visualization technique, breathing directly into each point of discomfort in your body; delivering oxygen and healing energy and removing all stress and anxiety.

- Bring your awareness now to the center of your forehead. Visualize the air entering your body here through imaginary nostrils. See the oxygen- and life-force-rich air swirling around, dissolving any tension behind the eyes and in all the muscles of your face. As you exhale, imagine all the stress and tension being carried away and released.

- Now bring your attention to the crown of your head where a small pair of nostrils is breathing in nutrient-rich oxygen and *prana*. Visualize this breath as a soft white mist, swirling down through the top of your head and spreading across your face, neck, shoulders, arms, chest, back, buttocks, thighs, knees, calves, feet and right down to your toes. Continue to breathe in and out until this white mist is filling your body from head to toe. As you breathe in and out, let this white mist flow all the way down your spine and out again. Visualize this mist swirling around your body taking away all remaining stress or tension. Allow yourself to experience the calmness and vitality this exercise can bring to you.

- Then when you are ready, begin to breathe normally. Give your body a stretch and slowly open your eyes. Allow yourself a few moments to reorient yourself before getting up. Be aware that this feeling of well-being will remain with you for the rest of the day.

ACKNOWLEDGMENTS

I'd like to acknowledge and thank the more than 700 of my students and 25 teachers whose experiences have helped me to fine-tune and hone T5T into the powerful program it is today.

My heartfelt gratitude and respect to the following health practitioners for their contributions to the physical development of T5T: Susie Lapin and Catherine Kernot, physiotherapists; Gina Richter, Pilates NY instructor; Tracey Stewart, Feldenkrais practitioner; Mathew Jennings and Libby Ross, osteopaths, Branko Kristevic, chiropractor; and Natalie Wareham, occupational health practitioner.

For helping bring this book to life my thanks go to the following people.

Michael Grant White, Breathing Development Expert of Optimal Breathing and www.breathing.com, who generously acted as a sounding board and gave advice regarding the breathing practices in T5T.

Martin Moroney, NLP master practitioner, corporate trainer and business coach of www.corporatefuturing.com.au, who tailored the NLP outcome process for T5T in Get Clear on What You Want.

Robyn Gilbey, my previous business partner who helped me get the business part of T5T up and going, and supported my efforts; and Chris Gilbey, who not only gave his time and advice, but introduced me to my literary agent, Mary Cunnane. Both Robyn and Chris are also long-term devoted T5T practitioners and friends.

Mary Cunnane, my agent, who really got behind me and continues to do so daily. It was Mary's inspiration to use the abbreviation (T5T) for what we used colloquially to refer to as The Five Tibetan Rites.

Julie Gibbs, and her staff at Penguin, who "put me through my paces" before becoming my "dream publisher." I have felt a true teamwork and absolute commitment in bringing this project into being.

My editor, Susan McLeish, who amazed me with her total grasp of T5T. Her everyday calmness and clarity under pressure were also inspirational. Susan was there for me in every possible way.

John Canty of Penguin Books—along with photo-shoot director Gayna Murphy and photographer Steve Murray—whose creative skills in the presentation of T5T really matched my hopes for it.

Aliza Fogelson, my editor at Clarkson Potter, who helped me through some harrowing deadlines and remained open to all my suggestions (and last-minute changes), as well as contributing her own valuable insights. The result is an even better book!

Peter McGuigan from Sanford J. Greenburger Associates, my agent in New York, whose inside knowledge, contacts and professionalism found me the ideal U.S. publisher, whose goals match my own.

Elise Green, my daughter Tess's best friend and T5T's model. You are truly stunning both in and out!

Atma Saraswati, accredited yoga teacher, who generously checked through my final proofs.

And finally, with great respect I acknowledge the lineage of teachers from whom these Rites originated, who would have tried and tested them throughout the centuries; I salute and honour you.

Private Tuition/Workshops/Corporate Groups/Teacher Training

Please visit our website, www.T5T.com, and blog, www.thefivetibetans.blogspot.com, for further tips, articles and information to assist you in your T5T practice.

For information on the T5T teacher training program please email teachertraining@T5T.com

Alternatively, you can contact us at PO Box 818, Avalon, NSW 2107, Australia.

Ancient and Contemporary Tibet

The original developers of The Five Tibetan Rules of Rejuvenation will probably never be discovered. When China invaded Tibet in the 1950s, they destroyed numerous monasteries, ancient spiritual texts and sacred images, and most likely with them the chance of discovering the true source of the Rites. Out of 6,259 monasteries and nunneries in the whole of Tibet, only eight remain undestroyed. (Source: Dept. of Culture & Religion, Tibetan Government-In-Exile)

The Dalai Lama and some 10,000 Tibetans fled Tibet in 1959 and settled in India, Nepal, Bhutan and elsewhere. Since then 100,000 Tibetans have been compelled to leave their homeland and live in exile. The Dalai Lama continues to maintain the Tibetan Government-in-exile from his base in Dharamsala, in northwest India.

If you would like to know more about Tibet or provide assistance in any way to help modern Tibetans maintain their ancient spiritual practices, please see the following:

Dalai Lama

His Holiness the 14th Dalai Lama, Tenzin Gyatso, is both the head of state and the spiritual leader of Tibet. He was awarded the Nobel Peace Prize in 1989 for his nonviolent struggle for the liberation of Tibet.

For information, email: info@dalailama.com
Website: http://www.dalailama.com

The Office of His Holiness the Dalai Lama
Thekchen Choeling
P.O. McLeod Ganj
Dharamsala H.P. 176219
India
Email: ohhdl@dalailama.com

Tibet House

Tibet House preserves and maintains Tibet's ancient culture and makes it available to others through art, photography, exhibitions, concerts and Tibetan Studies Programs, which include open meditation sessions and instruction, retreats, other spiritual practices and educational classes.

Tibet House Cultural Centre
22 West 15th Street (between 5th & 6th Ave.)
New York, New York 10011
General Information: (212) 807-0563
Website: http://www.tibethouse.org

A percentage of the monies received by the author in connection with this book is being donated to the Gyuto monks and Gyuto Tantric University in India—one of the few remaining places where the ancient, sacred Tibetan teachings are available.

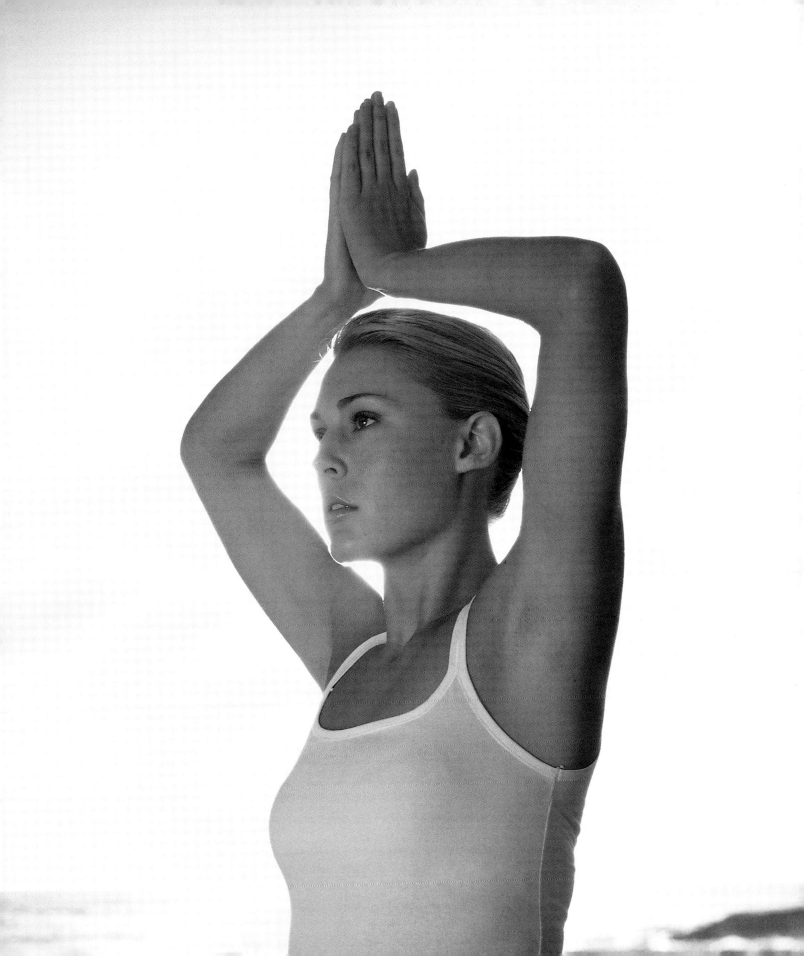

FURTHER READING

Breathing for health and vitality

Grant White, Michael, *Secrets of Optimal Natural Breathing Manual*, USA, 2004. (DVDs and audio cassettes available from Michael Grant White's website www.breathing. com) Mike is a very experienced breathing practitioner and teacher who has helped numerous people improve their breathing, Michael was very generous with his knowledge and ideas for the breathing sections of T5T.

Lewis, Dennis, *Free Your Breath, Free Your Life: How Conscious Breathing Can Relieve Stress, Increase Vitality and Help You Live More Fully*, Shambhala Publications, Boston, 2004. Easy to follow and understand, this book offers information and exercises for improving your breathing.

Farhi, Donna, *The Breathing Book: Vitality & Good Health Through Essential Breath Work*, Henry Holt & Company, New York, 1996. Focuses on relearning the deep, smooth, easy breath we had as children. With good illustrations and well-written text, this book is easy to understand and follow.

Fried, Robert, *Breathe Well, Be Well: A Program to Relieve Stress, Anxiety, Asthma, Hypertension, Migraine, and Other Disorders for Better Health*, John Wiley & Sons, USA, 1999. Written for laymen by a world-renowned expert in the treatment of stress and anxiety—Dr. Fried is professor of biopsychology and head of the respiratory psychophysiology laboratory at Hunter College, New York.

The Five Tibetan Rites of Rejuvenation

Kelder, Peter, *The Eye of Revelation*, Borderland Sciences Research Foundation, 1990 (first published in 1939). The original story of how the Rites were discovered and brought to the West.

Kelder, Peter, *Ancient Secret of the Fountain of Youth by Peter Kelder*, Volume I, Bantam Doubleday Dell Publishing Group (first published by Harbor Press, Gig Harbor, USA, 1985, reprinted 1989, 1998). The original story of how the Rites were discovered and brought to the West. Simple text with limited illustrations.

Kelder, Peter, *Ancient Secret of the Fountain of Youth by Peter Kelder*, Volume II, Bantam Doubleday Dell Publishing Group (first published by Harbor Press, Gig Harbor, USA, 1999). A companion book to Volume I, including insights on how the Rites work, people's experiences and diet suggestions.

Kilham, Christopher S., *The Five Tibetans: Five Dynamic Exercises for Health, Energy, and Personal Power*, Inner Traditions International (first published by Healing Art Press, USA, 1994.) Eloquent yet simple explanation of the Five Rites with basic instruction on kundalini meditation, chakras, relaxation and breathing.

Fusion of Pilates and yoga

Everett, Jill, *Pilates + Yoga*, Carlton Books, London, 2003. Clear, uncomplicated explanations with useful illustrations. A chiropractor's comments are included giving the benefits of, and cautions about, each posture.

Robinson, Lynne & Nappier, Howard, *Intelligent Exercise with Pilates & Yoga*, illustrated edition, MacMillan Pub. Ltd., UK, 2002. The shared knowledge of a leading Pilates teacher and a leading yoga teacher. Teaches you how to learn from and respect your body at all times.

Solomon, Louise, *Yogalates Total Body Toner: The Breakthrough Workout That Combines the Best Elements of Yoga and Pilates*, Virgin Books, Great Britain, 2003. Internationally acclaimed fusion of yoga with core stabilizing benefits of Pilates.

Yoga

Desikashar, TKV, *The Heart of Yoga: Developing a Personal Practice*, revised edition, Inner Traditions International, 1999. Desikashar, a world-renowned teacher, provides an in-depth but down-to-earth book on yoga and how to tailor it to the current health and needs of the individual.

Francina, Suza, *The New Yoga for People Over 50: A Comprehensive Guide for Midlife & Older Beginners*, Health Communications, USA, 1997.

Iyengar, BKS, *Light on Yoga: The Bible of Modern Yoga*, Thorsons, Great Britain, 2001 (first published by George Allen & Unwin, 1966). Shared knowledge of a great living teacher now in his 80s. Includes detailed descriptions and hundreds of illustrations.

Scaravelli, Vanda, *Awakening the Spine*, 2nd edition, HarperSanFrancisco, 1991. Vanda was a vibrant 83-year-old master teacher who came to yoga late in life. She taught "If it hurts, it's wrong!"

Flexibility

Laughlin, Kit, *Stretching & Flexibility*, Simon & Schuster (Australia), Australia, 2000. Very detailed yet well-described exercises to improve flexibility in every part of your body.

The Chakras and human energy system

Brennan, Barbara Ann, *Hands of Light: A Guide to Healing Through the Human Energy Field*, revised edition, Bantam, USA, 1988. Barbara Ann Brennan trained as a physicist and psychotherapist, and is now an expert on the human energy field. Her book teaches perceptual techniques for healing.

Leadbeater, Charles W., *The Chakras*, Theosophical Publishing House (first published by Cosmo Publications, USA, 2003). Originally published in the 1920s, a clairvoyant explains the human energy centers. Includes very good color illustrations of the chakras.

Myss, Caroline, *Anatomy of The Spirit: The Seven Stages of Power and Healing*, Three Rivers Press, USA, 1997. A medical intuitive and extensive researcher outlines how every illness corresponds to a pattern of attitudes and beliefs. Teaches you to see your body and spirit in a different way.

Singh Khalsa, Dr Dharma, *Meditation as Medicine: Activate the Power of Your Natural Healing Force*, Atria Books, 2002. A physician and yogi, Dr Dharma Singh Khalsa is an expert on anti-aging and medical meditation to overcome illness and improve health.

Mind–body connection

Dychtwald, Ken, *Bodymind*, revised edition, Pantheon Books, USA, 1986. Very engrossing and informative book about the connection between your body and mind. Good information about what your body shape and condition says about you.

Dziemidko, MD, Helen E., *The Complete Book of Energy Medicines: Choosing Your Path to Health*, Healing Arts Press, UK, 1999. A qualified doctor, homeopath, reflexologist and masseur gives an overview of the growing field of energy medicines in language that is easy to understand.

Noontil, Annette, *The Body Is the Barometer of the Soul, So Be Your Own Doctor*, 2nd edition, Rainbow Spirit, Australia, 1996. How to change your body by changing your thoughts.

Pert, Ph.D., Candace B., *Molecules of Emotion: The Science Behind Mind-Body Medicine*, Touchstone (first published by Scribner, USA, 1999). Amazing science and amazing personal story; will make you understand your world very differently.

Water

Browning, Tovi, *Gentle Miracles: Holistic Pulsing*, Global Embrace, Australia, 1990. Outlines the philosophy behind her development of Holistic Pulsing and gives detailed instructions on how to perform it.

Emoto, Masaru, *The Hidden Messages in Water*, By Beyond Words Publishing, USA, 2004. Absolutely amazing high-speed photographs of crystals formed in frozen water that show dramatic changes when specific, concentrated thoughts are directed toward them. This book will open your eyes as to how deeply water is connected to our individual and collective consciousness. Look under the heading for water on www.wellnessgoods.com to see some of these amazing images.

Other interesting titles

Chopra, Deepak, *Grow Younger Live Longer: Ten Steps to Reverse Aging*, Three Rivers Press, USA, 2002. Advice on how to develop a youthful mind, body and spirit.

Tolle, Eckhart, *The Power of Now, A Guide to Spiritual Enlightenment*, New World Library, USA, 1999. An excellent book on how to live a happier, more fulfilling life. Gives deep insights and practical advice on how to live in the moment.

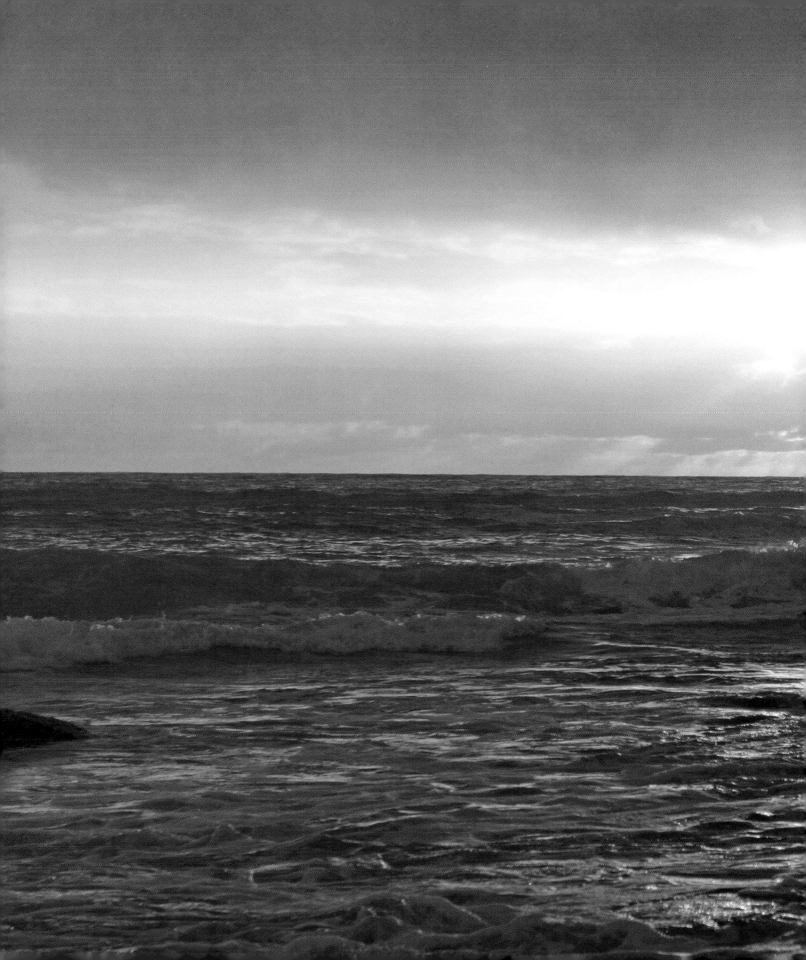

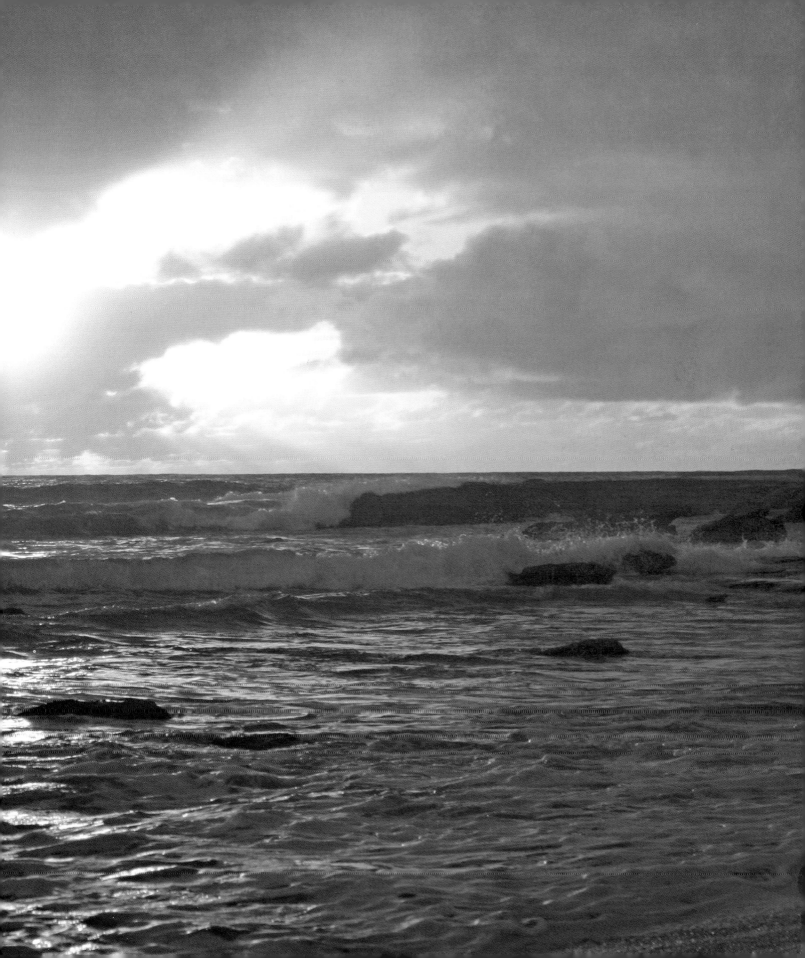